Digestive Diseases

Clinical Reviews

Formerly 'Survey of Digestive Diseases'
Founded in 1983 by T.S.N. Chen and R.K. Zetterman
Former Editor: S.R. Achem (1993–2000)

KARGER

Printed in Switzerland
on acid-free paper by
Reinhardt Druck, Basel

Appears quarterly:
1 volume per year
(4 issues)

General Information

Digestive Diseases

Publication data: 'Digestive Diseases' is published 4 times a year. Volume 20 with 4 issues appears in 2002.

Subscription rates: Subscriptions run for a full calendar year. Prices are given per volume.
Personal subscription:
Subscription + postage and handling
CHF 124.35 + CHF 19.20 Europe
CHF 124.35 + CHF 28.50 Overseas
USD 95.00 + USD 19.20
+ online subscription per volume:
CHF 39.– / USD 30.00
(Must be in the name of, billed to, and paid by an individual. Order must be marked 'personal subscription'.)
Institutional subscription:
Subscription + postage and handling
CHF 988.– + CHF 24.– Europe
CHF 988.– + CHF 35.60 Overseas
USD 760.00 + USD 24.00
+ online subscription per volume:
CHF 58.– / USD 45.00
Airmail postage: CHF 24.–, USD 20.00.
(Extra per volume.)
Discount subscription prices:
Please enquire about reduced rates for residents.

Microforms: Please direct all enquiries and orders to:
University Microfilms Inc.
300 North Zeeb Road, P.O. Box 1346
Ann Arbor, MI 48106-1346 (USA)

Subscription orders: Orders can be placed at agencies, bookstores, directly with the
Publisher S. Karger AG, P.O. Box,
CH–4009 Basel (Switzerland)
or with any of the following distributors:
Deutschland: S. Karger GmbH, Postfach
D–79095 Freiburg
France: Librairie Luginbühl
36, bd de Latour-Maubourg, F–75007 Paris
Great Britain, Ireland: S. Karger AG
4 Rickett Street
London SW6 1RU, UK
USA: S. Karger Publishers, Inc.
26 West Avon Road, P.O. Box 529
Farmington, CT 06085, USA
India, Bangladesh, Sri Lanka:
Panther Publishers Private Ltd.
33, First Main
Koramangala First Block
Bangalore 560 034, India
Japan: Karger Japan, Inc.
Yushima S Bld. 3F
4-2-3, Yushima, Bunkyo-ku
Tokyo 113-0034, Japan

Change of address: Both old and new address should be sent to the subscription source.

Single issues: Information can be obtained through the Publisher.

Advertising: Correspondence and rate requests should be addressed to the Publisher.

Bibliographic indices: This journal is regularly listed in bibliographic services, including *Current Contents*®.

Book Reviews: Books are accepted for review by special agreement.

Copying: This journal has been registered with the Copyright Clearance Center (CCC), as indicated by the code appearing on the first page of each article. For readers in the US, this code signals consent for copying of articles for personal or internal use, or for the personal or internal use of specific clients, provided that the stated fee is paid per copy directly to
Copyright Clearance Center Inc.
222 Rosewood Drive
Danvers, MA 01923 (USA).
A copy of the first page of the article must accompany payment. Consent does not extend to copying for general distribution, for promotion, for creating new works, or for resale. In these cases, specific written permission must be obtained from the copyright owner,
S. Karger AG, P.O. Box,
CH–4009 Basel (Switzerland).

KARGER

Fax +41 61 306 12 34
E-Mail karger@karger.ch
www.karger.com

The Journal Home Page is available at:
www.karger.com/journals/ddi

Digestive Diseases

Prevention and Progress in Management of Gastrointestinal Cancers

Editor

Peter Malfertheiner, Magdeburg

18 figures, 24 tables, 2002

KARGER

Basel · Freiburg · Paris · London · New York ·
New Delhi · Bangkok · Singapore · Tokyo · Sydney

S. Karger
Medical and Scientific Publishers
Basel · Freiburg · Paris · London
New York · New Delhi · Bangkok
Singapore · Tokyo · Sydney

Drug Dosage
The authors and the publisher have exerted every effort to ensure that drug selection and dosage set forth in this text are in accord with current recommendations and practice at the time of publication. However, in view of ongoing research, changes in government regulations, and the constant flow of information relating to drug therapy and drug reactions, the reader is urged to check the package insert for each drug for any change in indications and dosage and for added warnings and precautions. This is particularly important when the recommended agent is a new and/or infrequently employed drug.

Printed in Switzerland on acid-free paper by
Reinhardt Druck, Basel
ISBN 3–8055–7440–1

KARGER

Fax + 41 61 306 12 34
E-Mail karger@karger.ch
www.karger.com

Vol. 20, No. 1, 2002

Digestive Diseases

Contents

KARGER

Fax + 41 61 306 12 34
E-Mail karger@karger.ch
www.karger.com

Access to full text and tables of contents, including tentative ones for forthcoming issues:
www.karger.com/journals/ddi/ddi_bk.htm

Digestive Diseases

Dig Dis 2002;20:4

Editorial

The prevention of neoplastic disorders of the digestive system has moved ahead from a state of hopeful expectations in future possibilities to some current solid grounds of evidence based on interventions. Careful studies of familial genetic disorders, the identification of molecular targets, important epidemiological work revealing conditions for gastrointestinal cancer risks, and finally the appreciation of preneoplastic lesions has set an important stage in this field. The wide diffusion of standard diagnostic methods such as endoscopy as well as interventional techniques make it possible to offer new chances of maintaining or restoring health in patients that otherwise would incur a fate determining neoplastic disease. However, despite these achievements, to date we are facing an era that stands just at the beginning of an epochal revolution in the medical approaches to prevent and cure neoplastic disorders. The human genome sequence and the continuous development of molecular technologies will open more opportunities to define disease-promoting and determining genes in their interaction with the environment.

The dilemma is that in several circumstances the epidemiological and biological evidence will precede the required proof of confirmatory intervention studies by many years. This could become a concern if not handled with the appropriate sensitivity and alertness. In this issue of *Digestive Diseases* we have selected some of the key topics related to cancer prevention or new approaches to cancer therapy. Some strategies and approaches have already become part of our medical management (i.e. screening for colorectal cancer and polypectomy) and others find themselves in ongoing debate and need more specification (eradication of *H. pylori* for cancer prevention in risk individuals and populations at risk), some open fascinating future possibilities and some propose surgical interventions to prevent neoplasias in very selected cases.

We are indebted to all the authors for their invaluable contributions in providing an important update and further stimulation of our interest in this exploding field of medicine.

Peter Malfertheiner

KARGER

Fax + 41 61 306 12 34
E-Mail karger@karger.ch
www.karger.com

0257–2753/02/0201–0004$18.50/0

Accessible online at:
www.karger.com/journals/ddi

Review Article

Digestive Diseases

Dig Dis 2002;20:5–17

Photodynamic Therapy for Mucosal Esophageal Adenocarcinoma and Dysplastic Barrett's Esophagus

Herbert C. Wolfsen

Mayo Clinic, Jacksonville, Fla., USA

Key Words
Photodynamic therapy · Mucosal esophageal adenocarcinoma · Dysplastic Barrett's esophagus

Abstract
Photodynamic therapy is a novel endoscopic technique that combines a photosensitizer and laser light to destroy target cells. Photodynamic therapy has been used in Europe, North Africa and Japan to treat esophageal neoplasms and dysplastic Barrett's esophagus. This paper summarizes the available published experience of photodynamic therapy for the treatment of each esophageal cancer and Barrett's esophagus. These studies suggest that photodynamic therapy is a promising modality for esophageal mucosal disease. More long-term studies, however, are needed to document the efficacy of photodynamic therapy in reducing the morbidity and mortality from esophageal cancer for patients with high-grade dysplasia and early adenocarcinoma in Barrett's esophagus.

Introduction

Photodynamic therapy is used to treat cancerous or dysplastic conditions utilizing a photosensitizing agent and an external light source in the presence of oxygen. The photosensitizing agent is preferentially taken up into dysplastic or malignant cells and is activated by the application of light at a specific wavelength. The photosensitizer then achieves an excited stage, generating highly reactive oxygen species that result in cellular injury [1]. Photodynamic therapy has been demonstrated to destroy tissue based upon several effects [2] including: (a) direct cytotoxicity; (b) microvascular damage from platelet activation and thromboxane-induced vessel constriction and thrombus formation, probably mediated by nitric oxide [3]; (c) cytosolic and mitochondrial membrane damage with cytochrome C release, bcl-2 depletion and induction of apoptosis, and (d) release of inflammatory mediators that induce T-lymphocyte mediated cellular immune response [4–6]. While photodynamic therapy has been applied to a number of malignant and premalignant conditions, including cancers of the lung, breast, skin, ovary, throat, and larynx [7], most of the investigational work has focused on the esophagus and stomach [8, 9].

KARGER

Fax + 41 61 306 12 34
E-Mail karger@karger.ch
www.karger.com

0257–2753/02/0201–0005$18.50/0

Accessible online at:
www.karger.com/journals/ddi

Herbert C. Wolfsen, MD
Division of Gastroenterology and Hepatology, Mayo Clinic
4500 San Pablo Road
Jacksonville, FL 32224 (USA)
Tel. +1 904 953 2000, Fax +1 904 953 7260, E-Mail pdt@mayo.edu

Three basic elements are essential to the photodynamic reaction that is the basis of photodynamic therapy: a chemical photosensitizing agent, light, and oxygen. The photosensitizer is administered to the patient intravenously and is taken up and selectively retained by dysplastic and malignant cells. Forty-eight hours are allowed to pass before the patient is exposed to the light source, so that the drug is eliminated by normal tissues while still concentrated in abnormal cells. This enhances the relative specificity of the treatment [10]. Photodynamic therapy for diseases of the gastrointestinal tract requires endoscopic delivery of light to the target lesion(s). Since each photosensitizing compound has a unique absorption spectrum, light of a specific wavelength is administered to activate the photosensitizer, resulting in the formation of toxic oxygen metabolites, most likely singlet oxygen ($^1O_2$). In the gastrointestinal tract, the use of photodynamic therapy is particularly attractive since it allows a large area of epithelium to be treated with a low risk of perforation [10].

As mentioned above, the only photosensitizing agent that is commercially available and approved for clinical use in grastroenterologic photodynamic therapy is sodium porfimer. This agent is actually a mixture of several different porphyrin compounds. Seventy-five milligrams of the medication is diluted in 31.8 ml of normal saline or 5% dextrose, resulting in a drug concentration of 2.5 mg/ml. The drug is usually administered at a dose of 2 mg/kg [10]. It is not definitively known how the molecules of the photosensitizing agent localize in neoplastic cells. It has been observed that many photosensitizers have a high affinity for plasma low-density lipoproteins (LDL) and that tissues that preferentially take up photosensitizing drugs tend to actively express LDL receptors. Also, the target cells of photodynamic therapy usually are very metabolically active, but it is not known how this results in increased uptake of photosensitizing agents [11]. After sodium porfimer enters a cell, it is distributed throughout the cytoplasm and becomes tightly bound to mitochondrial membranes but other subcellular targets include lysosomes, Golgi apparatus, and the rough endoplasmic reticulum [12]. Later, more recently studied mechanisms of photodynamic therapy-induced cell death will be reviewed [2, 13].

After the photosensitizer has been concentrated in the target cells and released from the normal tissue, the mucosal target is exposed to light of a specific wavelength that is required to activate the drug. For sodium porfimer, red light at 630 m delivers a depth of tissue penetration of 5 to 8 mm. The depth of tissue penetration is dependent on the wavelength of light utilized and some investigators have used green light for more superficial tissue penetration [14].

Early Esophageal Adenocarcinoma

The standard treatment for operable patients with early-stage esophageal cancer is resection with curative intent [15]. A curative operation normally consists of an en bloc resection of the distal esophagus, proximal stomach, spleen and splenic artery, with regional lymph node dissection. Gastrointestinal continuity may be established through a gastric pull-up or colon interposition. The operative mortality rates vary from 2 to 12% and the morbidity is approximately 40–45%. The incidence of anastomotic strictures is 25%, even in experienced centers [16–18]. Another approach to a curative treatment for localized disease is external beam radiation. Several studies show that chemoradiation therapy is superior to radiation alone, at least in more advanced disease. Limited published data on radiation therapy for superficial esophageal cancer from Japan suggest that it can result in overall survival rates of about 38.7% as well as disease-specific 5-year survival rate of 71% [19]. Unfortunately, the complication rate was 15%, particularly in those with intraluminal radiation therapy (brachytherapy).

An alternative safe and effective non-surgical treatment is needed for patients who are poor surgical candidates due to comorbid disease. The endoscopic techniques that have been reported or are currently under evaluation for curative treatment of early esophageal cancer include photodynamic therapy [20–24], endoscopic mucosectomy/mucosal resection (EMR) [25–28] and laser photoablation [29, 30]. Yang et al. used Nd:YAG laser photoablation to eradicate early esophageal cancer [29] but tumor recurred in 27% of cases. The use of KTP lasers [30] and argon plasma coagulation has been limited to small pilot studies.

Photodynamic therapy using various photosensitizers is another highly promising endoscopic modality (table 1). Photodynamic therapy involves application of a photosensitizer drug through the oral or intravenous route. The drug localizes preferentially in much higher concentrations in dysplastic and malignant tissue than in normal cells. In the presence of oxygen, laser light at a specific wavelength activates the drug and results in a photochemical reaction that leads to selective tissue destruction. Photodynamic therapy has been applied to tumors in the esophagus, stomach, duodenum, bile duct,

Table 1. Photodynamic therapy for early esophageal cancer

Author, year, reference	Tumor histology	n	Photosensitizer	Response (%)
Overholt, 1997 [87]	ACA	7	Photofrin	7/7 (100)
Overholt, 1999 [82]	ACA	13	Photofrin	10/13 (77)
Wolfsen, 2002	ACA	12	Photofrin	11/12 (92)
Beejay, 2001 [88]	ACA	5	Photofrin	4/5 (80)
Etienne, 2001 [89]	ACA	11	Photofrin	11/11 (100)
Gossner, 1998 [20]	ACA	22	ALA	17/22 (77)
Gossner, 1999 [90, 91]	ACA	58	ALA w/THPC	36/58 (62)
Tan, 1999 [34]	ACA	12	ALA	2/12 (17)
Ackroyd, 1999 [92]	ACA	3	ALA	0/3 (0)
Sibille, 1995 [24]	SCC	37	Photofrin/HpD	30/37 (81)
Grosjean, 1998 [14, 93]	SCC	84	Photofrin/mTHPC	67/84 (80)
Hayata, 1996 [94]	SCC	33	HpD	32/33 (97)
Etienne, 2001 [89]	SCC	14	mTHPC	10/14 (71)
Savary, 1997 [41]	SCC	16	mTHPC	13/16 (81)
Savary, 1998 [23]	SCC	8	HpD	6/8 (75)
Savary, 1998 [23]	SCC	6	Photofrin	4/6 (67)
Savary, 1998 [23]	SCC	10	mTHPC	8/10 (80)
Messmann, 1997 [95]	SCC	6	HpD	6/6 (100)
McCaughan, 1996 [96]	SCC	3	HpD/Photofrin	N/A
Calzavara, 1990 [97]	SCC	21	HpD	11/21 (52)
Okunaka, 1990 [40]	SCC	6	HpD/Photofrin	11/21 (52)
Hayata, 1988 [98]	SCC	7	HpD	5/7 (71)
Tajiri, 1987 [99]	SCC	6	HpD	3/6 (50)
Fujimaki, 1986 [100]	SCC	15	HpD	10/15 (67)
Tian, 1985 [101]	SCC	13	HpD	12/13 (92)

lung, and other sites of the body, often in conjunction with other oncology treatments [31]. When applied in the gastrointestinal tract, the photosensitizer can be administered locally or intravenously.

One of the first clinical studies using aminolevulinic acid (ALA) photodynamic therapy was published by Regula in 1995 [32]. This series included 18 patients with esophageal cancer. While the ALA photodynamic therapy was found to be safe and effective with production of mucosal necrosis, neoplasms were not eliminated. Gossner et al., from Germany reported photodynamic therapy with 5-aminolevulinic acid (5-ALA) as a potential form of local mucosal ablative therapy for early esophageal cancer [30]. In this study, 32 patients [10 with HGD and 22 with mucosal adenocarcinomas ($T_{1m}N_0M_0$)] were staged by EUS [33]. Patients were then treated with oral 5-ALA activated by KTP dye laser-delivered light at 635 nm. Patients were followed for a mean of 9.9 months and required 2.2 photodynamic therapy treatments per patient on average. All patients took omeprazole at 20–80 mg/day. High-grade dysplasia was eliminated in all patients although Barrett's metaplasia was only partially re-epithelialized in 21 of 32 patients (68%) and in two patients nondysplastic Barrett's glands were detected under a neosquamous mucosal lining. Seventeen of 22 (77%) of cancers responded completely. However in 5 patients with tumors ≥2 mm in thickness the lesions persisted. These patients subsequently underwent curative treatment with mTHPC photodynamic therapy (3 patients) or esophagectomy (2 patients). Other ALA photodynamic therapy studies included a 12-patient series from Tan from the United Kingdom [34]. Of these patients, only 2 had successful disease eradication (1 patient with carcinoma in situ, 1 patient with an invasive cancer <1 cm in diameter). The other 10 patients (83%) had only superficial necrosis despite ALA doses up to 75 mg orally and repeated treatments up to 4 times. These and other studies confirm that mucosal necrosis is superficial and persistence of Barrett's glandular mucosa and particular subsquamous glandular mucosa occurs in a significant number of patients [35]. These and other data may indicate that ALA photodynamic therapy is best suited for patients with non-dysplastic Barrett's mucosa or Barrett's low grade dysplasia [36, 37]. Unfortunately, 5-ALA is not approved for use in the United States and the superficial treatment depth may be a limiting factor in its use for early cancer and Barrett's high-grade dysplasia [37, 38].

Photodynamic therapy using Photofrin® has been studied for the treatment of superficial early-stage esophageal carcinoma. Improved disease-specific survival rates point to the potentially curative efficacy of a local endoscopic treatment [20–24, 39–41]. In a study at the Mayo Clinic by Laukka et al., patients who had HGD or superficial cancer arising in BE and were ineligible for surgery were treated with photodynamic therapy using hematoporphyrin derivative (HPD) [42]. HPD is a less purified form of porfimer sodium (Photofrin, Axcan Pharma, Mont Saint-Hilaire, Canada) with approximately one-third the photosensitizer concentration. All patients received 3–4 mg/kg of HPD. Two days after injection, 630-nm laser light was administered at a dose of 200–250 J/cm^2 fiber at a power of 400 mW. All patients were admitted to the Mayo Clinic Research Center for treatment. Follow-up endoscopies were performed at 24 h after light administration and after 3 months. Eleven patients have undergone follow-up evaluations that have demonstrated elimination of the cancer in 3 of 5 patients (60%) and elimination of high-grade dysplasia in 5 of 6 patients (83%). The Barrett's segment decreased from 8 ± 1 cm at baseline to 2 ± 1 cm after PDT. Complete elimination of the whole segment of Barrett's esophagus occurred in 4/11 patients (36%). All patients experienced acute chest pain and nausea following PDT. Esophageal strictures developed within 1 month of PDT in 4 patients (20%) and all responded to dilation. Corti et al. also treated 48 patients with high-grade dysplasia or early carcinoma with HPD (energy dose 200–300 J/cm^2) and reported a complete response rate of 44% for this group [43]. The local recurrence rate on follow-up was 48% with an improved median overall survival in complete responders and 7% stricture rate.

Sibille et al. from France treated 123 patients with early esophageal cancers 0.5 to 4.0 cm in diameter (104 squamous cell, 19 adenocarcinoma) who were referred for nonsurgical treatment [24]. Eighty-two patients were staged by EUS; 61 had T_1 and 27 had T_2 cancers. All patients were evaluated with Lugol's dye or indigo carmine chromoscopy to evaluate endoscopic morphology. Tumors were classified as superficial (polypoid, flat, elevated, depressed, or ulcerated), protruding, ulcerative, or infiltrative. Patients were treated either with HPD or Photofrin using 630-nm light from a bare diffuser fiber and a light dose of 200 J/cm^2 of tumor area. Photodynamic therapy was applied alone in 56 patients or as part of a multimodality therapy including radiation and/or chemotherapy in the rest. Adverse effects included cutaneous photosensitization in 16 patients (13%) and none were severe. Esophageal strictures developed in 43 patients (35%), with 5 requiring multiple dilations. The overall complete tumor response was obtained in 87% of patients, with no significant difference between squamous (87.5%) or adenocarcinomas (89%). Interestingly, the complete response rate and survival rates were not different in patients treated with PDT alone (versus PDT as part of a multimodality treatment) or more invasive (T_2) tumors. Most importantly, local tumor recurrence occurred in 36% of all patients 12–18 months later and was significantly higher in the adenocarcinoma group compared to the squamous cell cancers (75 vs. 28.5%, respectively, $p < 0.001$). Tumor recurrences were retreated and complete response achieved in 83 and 62.5% of patients with recurrent squamous cell and adenocarcinoma, respectively. The overall 5-year survival for all patients was 25 ± 6%. The disease-specific survival rate was 74 ± 5%. Associated medical comorbidity was clearly associated with decreased survival. There was a trend for improved survival in the T_1 cancer (95%) compared to the T_2 cancer group (74%) but this was not statistically significant, probably due to small number of patients in this subgroup.

Doctor Overholt in Knoxville, Tenn., has reported on the first 100 patients with dysplasia and/or early carcinoma in BE treated with Photofrin-PDT and followed for a mean of 19 months (range 4–84) [22]. Of the 100 patients with BE, 13 patients had biopsy-proven, early esophageal carcinomas less than 1.5 cm in size (12 with T_1, 1 with T_2 cancer), 73 had high-grade dysplasia (HGD), and 14 patients had low-grade dysplasia (LGD). Patients with cancer were staged with standard EUS only. Photofrin was administered at a dose of 2.0 mg/kg with light application 48 h following injection. This drug dose is identical to that used for the palliative treatment of esophageal cancer. Light was administered with 3 different light delivery methods: 1.5–2.5 cm fiber optic diffuser (15 patients), fiber optic diffuser within a transparent 360°, 3 or 5 cm windowed, centering balloon (15 patients) and a combination of the 2 methods (25 patients). Total light dose varied from 100 to 300 J/cm, dependent on several factors: initial or follow-up light treatment, balloon/fiber optic combination, or fiber optic diffuser alone. Additional light was given as necessary, approximately 48 h after the first light application. Nd:YAG thermal ablation with a contact probe was given in 83 patients to destroy small, residual islands of Barrett's mucosa, generally at 3–6 months after photodynamic therapy. Follow-up endoscopies and biopsies were performed at one week and 3, 6, 9, and 12 months post photodynamic therapy. All patients received omeprazole, 20 mg twice a day for the first 3 months and then once a day. All patients received prophylactic intravenous hydration for 3 to 5 days following photodynamic therapy. All patients were treated as outpatients but 6 were hospitalized for adverse effects (1 heart transplant patient for cardiac monitoring, 3 patients for atrial fibrillation, and 2 patients for treatment of large pleural effusions).

Extensive mucosal ablation was observed in all patients following photodynamic therapy, with a reduction in the extent of the Barrett's mucosal by an estimated 75–80%. The treated glandular mucosa was replaced by squamous epithelium and was associated with a relocation of the squamo-columnar mucosal junction distally by an average of 6.0 cm (range 0–19 cm). Barrett's glandular mucosa was completely eliminated in 43 patients. Overall, for treated areas, 77% of cancer, 88% of high-grade dysplasia, and 92% of low-grade dysplasia segments were cleared by PDT and focal thermal ablation. Seventy-nine percent of patients had complete conversion of dysplastic or malignant Barrett's esophagus to normal squamous or nondysplastic Barrett's glandular mucosa. Cancer persistend in 3 of the 13 patients with cancer. One died of cryptococcal meningitis and sepsis without tumor progression; another underwent surgery 6 months post-PDT and had 1 regional lymph node with cancer; and the other patient was found to have cancer metastatic to celiac lymph nodes at surgery 3 months post-photodynamic therapy. The latter was felt to have been incorrectly staged by EUS. One patient with high-grade dysplasia developed a subsquamous cancer in a treated area. This was assumed to be present at the time of treatment (i.e. understaged by EUS and endoscopic biopsy) but not adequately destroyed. Retreatment with PDT resulted in a complete response with no recurrence for 2 years. Another 2 patients with high-grade dysplasia progressed to cancer detected by endoscopic biopsy but no cancer was detected at surgery (only high-grade dysplasia was present).

The most common post-PDT complication was the development of esophageal stricture in 34 patients (34%) that was severe in 11 patients and required multiple dilations [44]. Three patients developed atrial fibrillation requiring hospitalization. These patients received medical treatment and quickly returned to normal sinus rhythm with no myocardial injury. Pleural effusions were noted in most patients who underwent chest x-rays 48 h after treatment. All patients were asymptomatic with respect to pulmonary symptoms. Atrial fibrillation and the development of asymptomatic pleural effusions are felt to be the result of a local-regional inflammatory reaction. Four patients (4%) developed significant sunburn following PDT. There were no esophageal perforations and no 30-day mortality reported.

At the Mayo Clinic in Jacksonville, Florida, 40 patients have been treated with Photofrin® photodynamic therapy for dysplastic Barrett's esophagus including 12 patients with $T_1N_0M_0$ Barrett's adenocarcinoma. All patients had been evaluated with contrast-enhanced computed tomography of the chest and abdomen as well as standard and high-frequency catheter endosonography. A cardiothoracic surgeon had evaluated all patients and these patients either refused the operation or were not considered surgical candidates. After photodynamic therapy, we used the argon plasma coagulator (Erbe Medizintechnik, Tübingen, Germany) to thermoablate small residual areas of Barrett's glandular mucosa. Patients were followed every 3 to 6 months with an aggressive endoscopic surveillance program. Apparent complete photoablation of Barrett's mucosa and/or superficial neoplasm was documented in 39 of 40 cases at a median series follow-up of 19 months (range 2–47 months). Complications included symptomatic strictures in 10 patients, photosensitivity reactions in 7 patients, atrial fibrillation or recurrent congestive heart failure and self-limited esophageal perforation (1 patient each). Failure to ablate $T_1N_0M_0$ adenocarcinoma occurred in one patient.

These data indicate that photodynamic therapy is a very promising modality in the treatment of early esophageal cancer. Compared to the results of ALA photodynamic therapy, Photofrin photodynamic therapy produced deeper tissue necrosis and is seemingly much more effective in eradicating Barrett's glandular mucosa and early neoplasms [45]. The trade off is the higher incidence of strictures and prolonged photosensitization associated with Photofrin photodynamic therapy [8].

Barrett's Esophagus

Barrett's esophagus is a condition in which the normal stratified squamo-columnar epithelium or mucosa lining the distal esophagus is replaced over time by specialized (metaplastic) columnar epithelium [46–49]. It is characterized endoscopically by a red, velvet-like texture which contrasts sharply with the pale, glossy appearance of adjacent normal squamo-columnar epithelium. This process results in displacement into the distal esophagus of the squamo-columnar (SC) mucosal junction (or Z-line) from the gastroesophageal (GE) junction. The new SC junction may be circumferential or irregular or appear as finger-like projections or isolated islands of columnar epithelium, or any combination of these forms [50, 51]. While Barrett's esophagus is clearly recognizable at endoscopy, diagnosis of dysplasia or early carcinoma can only be made from histological review of multiple biopsies. Barrett's esophagus develops when the normal squamo-columnar epithelium lining the distal esophagus is replaced by metaplastic columnar epithelium during the process of healing after a chronic injury to the esophageal mucosa. In most patients with Barrett's esophagus, chronic gastroesophageal reflux is responsible for providing the abnormal environment leading to this injury. Patients with Barrett's esophagus are at risk for development of dysplasia. Continued reflex causes initially mild (low-grade), and later severe (high-grade) dysplasia. On a background of a dysplastic epithelium, esophageal adenocarcinoma may develop [49]. Dysplasia in Barrett's esophagus has, therefore, been identified as a premalignant condition culminating in esophageal adenocarcinoma [52, 53].

The estimated risk of adenocarcinoma for patients with Barrett's esophagus varies considerably in published literature. Risk is frequently described as the incidence of adenocarcinoma in Barrett's esophagus patients followed for a number of years of follow-up. Endoscopic surveillance studies show the development of adenocarcinoma varies from 1 case in 16 to 1 case in 41 patients-years of follow-up, or 30 to 169 times greater than the general population [48]. While the incidence of squamous cell carcinoma of the esophagus is decreasing, adenocarcinoma of the lower esophagus is one of the malignancies showing a rapid increase in incidence in the US [54].

There is substantial debate concerning the management of the patient whose endoscopic biopsies show high-grade dysplasia without adenocarcinoma. Some authors recommend esophagectomy for these patients [49, 54] while others advocate continued endoscopic surveillance until biopsy evidence of esophageal cancer is found [51, 52, 55–57]. The proponents of esophagectomy argue that the high prevalence of associated invasive carcinoma in patients with high-grade dysplasia justifies resection. The basis for this concern are reports indicating that invasive carcinoma was found in 33 to 74% of patients who had esophagectomy for persistent high-grade dysplasia [48, 49, 57]. The proponents of endoscopic surveillance, however, argue that only 20 to 26% of high-grade dysplasia patients develop adenocarcinoma after a median follow-up of 12 to 24 months [58, 59], and that up to 80% of patients with high-grade dysplasia did not develop adenocarcinoma over a follow-up period of 156 patient-years [58]. Those patients who do progress to adenocarcinoma can be detected at a curative stage with a rigorous, systemic endoscopic biopsy protocol [58, 59]. Pallay et al. have recommended that the finding of high-grade dysplasia be confirmed by another expert pathologist and a repeat endoscopic examination after at least 1 month before esophagectomy is considered [60]. Even with this approach, approximately half of the patients receive a prophylactic esophagectomy, a procedure which has a substantial mortality of 3 to 7% and significant morbidity of 15 to 32% in the most recent series [61]. The Mayo Clinic group has reported a correlation of the density of highly dysplastic glands (focal vs. diffuse) that seemed to predict the development of invasive cancer in their Barrett's high-grade dysplasia patients [53]. Schnell et al. [57] have also reported extraordinary results in 1,099 patients with Barrett's esophagus followed with endoscopic surveillance for 5 to 7 years. This study found an incidence of progression in patients with Barrett's high-grade dysplasia to invasive cancer in only 16%, despite nearly 80% of patients being diagnosed with dysplasia at some point in the study. The use of a single pathologist is a weakness of the study [62], and the use of a year-long intensive endoscopy screening pre-surveillance protocol also limits the usefulness of the study [52].

Medical therapy with long-term acid suppression by omeprazole has only produced partial regression of non-dysplastic Barrett's epithelium [63, 64]. There is no evidence of regression of dysplasia with medical therapy. However, it is possible that progression of dysplasia to cancer may be delayed by the use of medical therapy such as high-dose omeprazole. Some authors have reported the disappearance of high-grade dysplasia on repeated endoscopic biopsies in up to 27% of patients [65, 66], although this could be attributed either to sampling error, or to the removal of high-grade dysplasia during the multiple biopsy procedures. Reports of several endoscopic ablation techniques, such as the thermal Nd:YAG laser, argon and KTP lasers, and multipolar electrocoagulation have all shown regression and in some cases total reversal of Barrett's esophagus [67–69]. However, none of these techniques have been studied in a randomized trail in patients with high-grade dysplasia to prove their efficacy in completely eradicating high-grade dysplasia, and thus decreas-

Table 2. Photodynamic therapy for Barrett's esophagus (BE) with high grade dysplasia (HGD)

Author	n	Photosensitizer	Subsquamous Barrett's %	BE elimination %	HGD elimination %	Stricture rate %	Use of fiber centering device?	Series average follow-up, months
PHO-BAR*	132	Photofrin	N/A	41	72	36	yes	12
Overholt [22]	73	Photofrin	6	44	88	34	yes	19
Wolfsen, 2002	28	Photofrin	0	50	100	25	no	19
Beejay [88]	13	Photofrin	N/A	61	100	55	yes	30
Wang [102]	26	HpD	4	35	88	27	no	N/A
Gossner [90, 91]	14	ALA/mTHPC	N/A	N/A	100	N/A	yes	N/A
Gossner [20]	10	ALA	20	0	100	0	yes	9.9
Barr [76]	5	ALA	40	0	100	0	yes	26–44
Ackroyd [92]	4	ALA	N/A	25	100	0	yes	28

* Thirty-site, international multi-center randomized control trial with 69 observation patients treated with omeprazole only, presented by Doctor Overholt at the International Photodynamic Association 8th World Congress of Photodynamic Medicine, Vancouver, Canada, June 5–9, 2001.

ing the risk of progression to cancer compared to a control group.

A minimally invasive treatment alternative for patients with Barrett's esophagus and dysplasia is clearly needed. Endoscopic techniques that have been utilized for ablation of Barrett's disease include thermal ablation using Nd:YAG laser [67], KTP laser [30, 70], and argon beam coagulation [71]. In a study of 16 patients with Barrett's without dysplasia treated with KTP laser, squamous epithelialization was noted in each case. In 11 patients (69%), though, Barrett's glands were noted to underlie the squamous mucosa, and in 9 patients squamous metaplasia was seen within Barrett's glands. In another report of 10 patients with Barrett's mucosa, complete mucosa ablation was noted in each case, but again, glandular mucosa was detected beneath the neosquamous lining [30]. In a study of 24 patients with Barrett's esophagus including 6 patients with dysplasia, argon plasma coagulation treatment produced complete ablation of Barrett's epithelium was noted in 13 patients [71]. The results, however, required repeated treatments (median 2; range 1–7) and 2 esophageal perforations (1 fatal) occurred. Compared to these non-selective 'point and shoot' techniques, photoablation with photodynamic therapy represents an attractive treatment alternative [72]. A summary of the pertinent photodynamic therapy studies in patients treated for Barrett's esophagus with high-grade dysplasia is presented in table 2.

In the United Kingdom and Europe, much work has focused on photodynamic therapy using 5-aminolevulinic acid in these patients [73, 74]. Gossner et al. used 5-aminolevulinic acid photodynamic therapy in 10 patients with Barrett's disease and high-grade dysplasia. Using high-dose gastric acid suppression post-treatment, they were able to demonstrate complete ablation of dysplastic tissue at a follow-up of nearly 10 months [30, 75]. Barr et al. published a small series of 5 patients with Barrett's patients with high-grade dysplasia [76]. Only one patient had complete Barrett's ablation and regrowth of squamous mucosa. Two patients had nondysplastic Barrett's beneath the neo-squamous mucosa. The other two patients had squamous mucosa developed within glands of nondysplastic Barrett's mucosa. Whether these glands are 'protected' by a squamous lining or more likely to develop neoplastic degeneration, only time will tell.

The most important study undertaken to date using aminolevulinic acid photodynamic therapy for dysplastic Barrett's esophagus has come from the University of Sheffield, England, in which 36 patients with Barrett's esophagus and low-grade dysplasia were randomized to receive either 30 mg/kg of aminolevulinic acid taken orally or observation [77]. Four or 6 h later, patients randomized to photodynamic therapy underwent light treatment using a copper vapor laser to produce green light at 514 nm wavelength and a 14-mm diameter clear Perspex cylindrical-shaped light diffuser with central channel housing the laser fiber diffuser in order to achieve uniform light dosimetry. Patients were examined with endoscopy and biopsy ever 1, 6, 12, and 24 months after photodynamic therapy. In the photodynamic therapy group, 4 h later, up to 6 cm Barrett's segment length per patient was then treated. Responses after ALA photodynamic therapy were seen in 16 of 18 (89%) in the ALA-photodynamic therapy group with a 30% median decrease in the area of Barrett's glandular mucosa (range 0 to 60%). Biopsies of the neosquamous areas found no squamous dysplasia or underlying columnar epithelium, although a rigorous biopsy protocol was not used. Barrett's glandular mucosa was not eliminated, however, in any of the photodynamic therapy related patients. These persistent areas of Barrett's epithelium were found to be free of dysplasia although there was also clearance of dysplasia in one-third of the patients in the observation group. In the observation group, no median decrease in Barrett's segment length was noted. Ablated areas of Barrett's in the ALA-photodynamic therapy group remained normal over the 24-month study follow-up period, and no dysplasia was found in areas where Barrett's mucosa remained. In the placebo group, low-grade dysplasia persisted in 12/18 patients (67%) over the 24-month study follow-up. Side effects were limited to the expected mediastinitis that required medical treatment in only 3 of 18 (17%) patients. One patient experienced a mild phototoxic reaction, but no esophageal strictures or dysphagia was noted after ALA-photodynamic therapy. These investigators are now reportedly randomizing patients to receive photodynamic therapy using higher doses of ALA (30 and 60 mg/kg) to try to produce more effective photoablation [45].

While these studies have demonstrated the safety and feasibility of ALA photodynamic therapy, concerns remain regarding the limited tissue penetration and high rate of subsquamous glandular epithelium in patients treated for Barrett's high-grade dysplasia and ineffective photoablation in patients treated for Barrett's low-grade dysplasia [37, 72]. While some ALA photodynamic therapy investigators have identified the importance of complete Barrett's ablation [36], others have suggested that buried glandular mucosa may prevent exposure to harmful refluxates and reduce the risk of potential malignant change [78, 79]. Since there are reports of cancers developing from glandular mucosa underlying squamous mucosa [22, 80] this issue will remain an important one and long-term follow-up of patients who have undergone ablation treatment [22, 35, 36, 80–82]. The use of interrupted light doses may be able to improve mucosal necrosis [83].

In controlled clinical trials, porfimer sodium photodynamic therapy has been shown to be effective for the reduction of obstruction and palliation of dysphagia in patients with complete or partial esophageal obstructions due to tumor. It has also shown promise as a treatment for superficial early-stage esophageal carcinoma where improved disease-specific survival rates point to the potentially curative efficacy of a local endoscopic treatment [24, 39, 84–86]. There are two ongoing studies on the Mayo Clinic. One is a controlled trial of low-dose photodynamic therapy for the treatment of Barrett's esophagus and the other is a single arm study of the treatment of high-grade dysplasia or cancer within Barrett's esophagus. Of the 75 patients enrolled in the controlled trial, 20 patients were prospectively randomly selected as the control group (omeprazole alone) [84–86]. Among the 55 photodynamic therapy-treated patients, 32 patients also had low-grade dysplasia in addition to Barrett's esophagus. Patients in the photodynamic therapy group received hematoporphyrin derivative at a dose of 1.5 to 2.0 mg/kg plus omeprazole. This is a low dose of the photosensitizer hematoporphyrin derivative that is a less purified form of porfimer sodium with approximately one-third of the photosensitizer concentration. Two days after hematoporphyrin derivative injection, 630-nm laser light was administered at a dose of 175 to 275 J/cm fiber using a 1.5–2.5 cm cylindrical diffusing fiber at a power of 400 mW. Follow-up endoscopy and biopsies were performed at 6-month intervals. All treatment was administered on an outpatient basis. The length of the Barrett's segment was reduced significantly from 7 ± 1 to 4 ± 1 cm ($p < 0.001$) following photodynamic therapy, but was unchanged ($p > 0.05$) in the control group. Seven patients (13%) in the photodynamic therapy group had their Barrett's segment eliminated entirely. Overall, histological grade significantly improved after photodynamic therapy, primary due to elimination of Barrett's ($p < 0.05$). The development of strictures was not reported to occur, although sunburn and odynophagia were common. In the other study conducted at the Mayo Clinic, results have been reported for 11 patients. Twenty patients had high-grade dysplasia or superficial cancer and were ineligible for surgery. All patients received 3–4 mg/kg of HPD. Two days after injection, 630-nm laser light was administered at a dose of 200–250 J/cm fiber at a power of 400 mW. All patients were admitted to the Mayo Clinic Research Center for treatment. Follow-up endoscopies were performed at 24 h after light administration and after 3 months. Eleven patients have undergone follow-up evaluations that have demonstrated elimination of the cancer in 3 of 5 patients (60%) and elimination of high-grade dysplasia in 5 of 6 (83%). the Barrett's segment decreased from 8 ± 1 cm at baseline to 2 ± 1 cm after photodynamic therapy. Complete elimination of the whole segment of Barrett's esophagus occurred in 4 of 11 patients (36%). All patients experienced acute chest pain and nausea following photodynamic therapy. Esophageal strictures developed within 1 month of photodynamic therapy in 4 patients (20%) and all responded to dilation. Previous studies from this group included an attempt to use lower doses of hematoporphyrin derivative for photodynamic therapy but results were limited [42].

The largest studies conducted to date of porfimer sodium for the treatment of dysplasia and/or carcinoma in Barrett's esophagus are currently ongoing at the Thompson Cancer Survival Center in Knoxville, Tenn., USA, [39]. Approximately 120 patients had been treated at the time of writing. In a recent update of the first study, Doctor Bergein Overholt reports on 55 patients with dysplasia and/or early carcinoma in Barrett's esophagus treated with photodynamic therapy using profimer sodium and followed for a minimum of 6 months. Of the 55 patients with Barrett's esophagus, 18 patients had biopsy-proven early esophageal carcinomas less than 1.5 cm in size, 25 had high-grade dysplasia and 12 patients had low-grade dysplasia. Porfimer sodium was administered at a dose of 2.0 mg/kg with light application 48 h following injection. This drug dose is identical to that used for the palliative treatment of esophageal cancer. Light was administered with 3 different light delivery methods: 1.5–2.5 cm fiber optic diffuser (15 patients), fiber optic diffuser within a transparent 360°, 3 or 5 cm windowed, centering balloon (15 patients) and a combination of the 2 methods (25 patients). Total light dose varied from 100 to 300 J/cm, dependent on several factors: initial or follow-up light treatment, balloon/fiber optic combination; or fiber optic diffuser alone. Additional light was given as necessary, approximately 48 h after the first light application. Nd:YAG thermal ablation was given in 28 patients to destroy small, residual islands of Barrett's mucosa, generally at 3–6 months after photodynamic therapy. Follow-up endoscopies and biopsies were performed at one week and 3, 6, 9, and 12 months post-photodynamic therapy. All patients received omeprazole, 20 mg twice a day for the first 3 months and then once a day. All but one patient were treated as outpatients. All patients received prophylactic intravenous hydration for 5 days following photodynamic therapy. Forty-two patients received 1 course, 10 patients received 2 courses, and 3 patients received 3 courses of photodynamic therapy. Duration of follow-up ranged from 6 to 66 months.

Extensive mucosal ablation was observed in all patients following photodynamic therapy, with a reduction in the extent of the Barrett's mucosa by an estimated 75–80%. The treated glandular mucosa was replaced by squamo-columnar epithelium and was associated with a relocation of the squamo-columnar mucosal junction distally in 24 patients by an average of 6.4 cm. All 18 patients with superficial esophageal carcinomas demonstrated biopsy-negative complete responses after photodynamic therapy. In 25 patients with high-grade dysplasia, it was abolished in 22. Therefore, of 43 patients with high-grade dysplasia and/or adenocarcinoma, 40 patients (93%) had ablation of their high-grade dysplasia/cancer following photodynamic therapy. Eleven of 12 patients treated for low-grade dysplasia had no dysplasia on follow-up. Esophageal strictures developed in 29 patients (53%) and were severe in 4 patients requiring multiple dilations. Two patients developed atrial fibrillation requiring hospitalization. Both patients received medical treatment and quickly returned to normal sinus rhythm with no myocardial injury. Pleural effusions were noted in most patients who underwent chest x-rays 48 h after treatment. All patients were asymptomatic with respect to pulmonary symptoms. Atrial fibrillation and the development of asymptomatic pleural effusions are thought to be the result of a local-regional inflammatory reaction. Four patients developed severe photosensitivity reactions following photodynamic therapy.

As reviewed previously, Doctor Overholt has updated and expanded this series [22, 44]. He has also recently presented long-term follow-up data on 74 patients treated with photodynamic therapy (mean follow-up 60 months, range 41–132 months). Following photodynamic therapy, the length of the Barrett's mucosa decreased by a mean of 7.2 cm (range 0–19 cm). Sixty of 62 patients experienced elimination of their high-grade dysplasia (97%). Three patients (5%) developed subsquamous adenocarcinoma compared to the expected incidence of 16–31 cases usually found in high-grade dysplasia patients (25–50%). In high-grade dysplasia patients, subsquamous, non-dysplastic metaplastic epithelium was found in 4 patients (5%). Strictures occurred in 18% with one photodynamic therapy treatment and 50% with two treatments for an overall stricture rate of 30%. Porfimer sodium photodynamic therapy then, with continuous Omeprazole therapy, reduces the length of Barrett's glandular mucosa, eliminates high-grade dysplasia in 97% of cases and reduces the expected incidence of esophageal cancer.

Results of a multicenter partially blinded, randomized study of the efficacy of photodynamic therapy using porfimer sodium for ablation of high-grade dysplasia Barrett's esophagus were presented at the 8th congress of Photodynamic Medicine in Vancouver, Canada, June 2001. Patients were randomized to observation with omeprazole 20 mg per day (n = 70) or photodynamic therapy using 2 mg/kg porfimer sodium and reflective, centering balloon device (n = 138). A centralized pathology laboratory reviewed specimens obtained at endoscopy every 3 months after photodynamic therapy (4 quadrant biopsies every 2 cm Barrett's segment length). At 6 months post-photodynamic therapy, high-grade dysplasia was eliminated in 80% of photodynamic therapy patients compared to 40% in the observation group. At a mean follow-up of 12.1 months, disease progression was noted in 39% of the observation group compared with 17% of the photodynamic therapy group. The most common adverse event was the development of esophageal stricture which occurred in 12.2% of patients after their first course of photodynamic therapy and 38% of patients overall. The group treated with porfimer sodium photodynamic therapy not only had effective elimination of areas with high-grade dysplasia but also incurred a 50% reduction in the rate of progression to adenocarcinoma.

At the Mayo Clinic in Jacksonville, Fla., USA, 28 patients with high-grade dysplasia in Barrett's esophagus who had been referred for PDT either because they refused esophagectomy or because they had been deemed poor candidates for the operation. Initial evaluation included computed tomography (CT) as well as standard and high frequency catheter endosonography (EUS). All patients were maintained on high-dose proton pump inhibitors. Follow-up endoscopy was performed in 4–6 weeks after PDT with ablation of any residual glandular mucosa using the argon plasma coagulator. Patients were then followed indefinitely every 3–6 months with CT, EUS and endoscopic surveillance. The median series follow-up was 19 months (range 2–47 months). Apparent complete photoablation of Barrett's mucosa after PDT and argon plasma thermoablation was documented in 39 of 40 cases. Complications included symptomatic strictures (10 patients), photosensitivity reactions (7 patients) atrial fibrillation or recurrent congestive heart failure, and self-limited esophageal perforation (1 patient each). Photodynamic therapy using porfimer sodium, then, appeared to eradicate dysplastic Barrett's mucosa in all 28 of these patients during a limited period of follow-up (median duration 19 months). There were no deaths but serious complications occurred.

Conclusions

These studies suggest that PDT is a promising modality for esophageal mucosal disease. However, long-term studies are needed to document the efficacy of PDT in reducing the morbidity and mortality from esophageal cancer for patients with high-grade dysplasia and early adenocarcinoma in Barrett's esophagus. The highly anticipated results of the multicenter controlled trial of profimer sodium photodynamic therapy to confirm these results and perhaps pave the way to an additional photodynamic therapy usage approval for Barrett's glandular mucosa with high-grade dysplasia. Regardless of method utilized to ablate Barrett's high-grade dysplasia, long-term endoscopic surveillance will remain necessary. This is particularly so, since follow-up histologic studies have documented persistence of pre-malignant genetic alteration after photodynamic therapy [35, 81].

References

1 Dougherty TJ, Gomer CJ, Henderson BW, Jori G, Kessel D, Korbelik M, Moan J, Peng Q: Photodynamic therapy. J Natl Cancer Inst 1998;90:889–905.
2 Oleinick NL, Evans HH: The photobiology of photodynamic therapy: Cellular targets and mechanisms. Radiat Res 1998;150:s146–156.
3 Korbelik M, Parkins CS, Shibuya H, Cecic I, Stratford MR, Chaplin DJ: Nitric oxide production by tumour tissue: Impact on the response to photodynamic therapy. Br J Cancer 2000;82:1835–1843.
4 Hsi RA, Rosenthal DI, Glatstein E: Photodynamic therapy in the treatment of cancer: Current state of the art. Drugs 1999;57:725–734.
5 Luo Y, Kessel D: Initiation of apoptosis versus necrosis by photodynamic therapy with chloraluminum phthalocyanine. Photochem Photobiol 1997;66:479–483.
6 He J, Oleinick NL: Cell death mechanisms vary with photodynamic therapy dose and photosensitizer; in Cortese DA (ed): 5th International Photodynamic Association Biennial Meeting. Vol 2371. Amelia Island, FL: SPIE, 1995, pp 92–96.
7 Pass HI: Photodynamic therapy in oncology: Mechanisms and clinical use. J Natl Cancer Inst 1993;85:443–456.
8 Wolfsen HC: Photodynamic therapy in gastroenterology: Current status in year 2000. Endoscopy 2000;32:715–719.
9 Carruth JA: Clinical applications of photodynamic therapy. Int J Clin Pract 1998;52:39–42.
10 Wang K: Photodynamic therapy made simple. Clin Persp Gastroenterol 2001;March/April: 90–100.

11 Webber J, Herman M, Kessel D, Fromm D: Current concepts in gastrointestinal photodynamic therapy. Ann Surg 1999;230:12–23.
12 Kubba AK: Role of photodynamic therapy in the management of gastrointestinal cancer. Digestion 1999;60:1–10.
13 Xue LY, Chiu SM, Oleinick NL: Photochemical destruction of the Bcl-2 oncoprotein during photodynamic therapy with the phthalocyanine photosensitizer Pc 4. Oncogene 2001;20: 3420–3427.
14 Grosjean P, Wagnieres G, Fontolliert C, van den Bergh H, Monnier P: Clinical photodynamic therapy for superficial cancer in the oesophagus and the bronchi: 514 nm compared with 630 nm light irradiation after sensitization with Photofrin II. Br J Cancer 1998;77: 1989–1995.
15 Nguyen NT, Schauer P, Luketich JD: Minimally invasive eosphagectomy for Barrett's esophagus with high-grade dysplasia. Surgery 2000; 127:284–290.
16 Peters JH, Bonavina L, Fleischer D, Greene FL, Hagen JA: Esophageal cancer: Surgical resection and adjuvant therapy. Contemporary Surgery 2001;57:15–21.
17 Thomas P, Doddoli C, Lienne P, Morati N, Thirion X, Garbe L, Giudicelli R, Fuentes P: Changing patterns and surgical results in adenocarcinoma of the oesophagus. Br J Surg 1997;84:119–125.
18 Wright TA: High-grade dysplasia in Barrett's oesophagus. Br J Surg 1997;84:760–766.
19 Okawa T, Tanaka M, Kita-Okawa M, Nishio M, Kikuchi Y, Shirato H, Yamada S, Asakawa H, Niibe H, Dokiya T, et al: Superficial esophageal cancer: Multicenter analysis of results of definitive radiation therapy in Japan. Radiology 1995;196:271–274.
20 Gossner L, Stolte M, Sroka R, Rick K, May A, Hahn EG, Ell C: Photodynamic ablation of high-grade dysplasia and early cancer in Barrett's esophagus by means of 5-aminolevulinic acid. Gastronenterology 1998;114:448–455.
21 Overholt B, Panjehpour M, Tefftellar E, Rose M: Photodynamic therapy for treatment of early adenocarcinoma in Barrett's esophagus. Gastrointest Endosc 1993;39:73–76.
22 Overholt BF, Panjehpour M, Haydek JM: Photodynamic therapy for Barrett's esophagus: Follow-up in 100 patients. Gastrointest Endosc 1999;49:1–7.
23 Savary JF, Grosjean P, Monnier P, Fontolliet C, Wagnieres G, Braichotte D, van den Bergh H: Photodynamic therapy of early squamous cell carcinomas of the esophagus: A review of 31 cases. Endoscopy 1998;30:258–265.
24 Sibille A, Lambert R, Souquet JC, Sabben G, Descos F: Long-term survival after photodynamic therapy for esophageal cancer. Gastroenterology 1995;108:337–344.
25 Ell C, May A, Gossner L, Guenter E, Mayer G: Endoscopic mucosectomy of early adenocarcinoma in patients with photodynamic therapy with Barrett's esophagus (abstract). Gastroenterology 1998;114:A589.
26 Fleischer DE, Wang GQ, Dawsey S, Tio TL, Newsome J, Kidwell J, Prifti S: Tissue band ligation followed by snare resection (band and snare): A new technique for tissue acquisition in the esophagus. Gastrointest Endosc 1996;44: 68–72.
27 Inoue H: Endoscopic mucosal resection for esophageal and gastric mucosal cancers. Can J Gastroenterol 1998;12:355–359.
28 Inoue H, Takeshita K, Hori H, Muraoka Y, Yoneshima H, Endo M: Endoscopic mucosal resection with a cap-fitted panendoscope for esophagus, stomach, and colon mucosal lesions. Gastrointest Endosc 1993;39:58–62.
29 Yang GR, Zhao LQ, Li SS, Qiu SL, Wang YM, Jia JH: Endoscopic Nd:YAG laser therapy in patients with early superficial carcinoma of the esophagus and the gastric cardia. Endoscopy 1994;26:681–685.
30 Gossner L, May A, Stolte M, Seitz G, Hang EG, Ell C: KTP laser destruction of dysplasia and early cancer in columnar-lined Barrett's esophagus. Gastrointest Endosc 1999;49:8–12.
31 Maier A, Woltsche M, Fell B, Prettenhofer U, Domej W, Roger GM, Pinter H, Smolle-Juttner FM: Local and systemic treatment in small cell carcinoma of the esophagus. Oncol Rep 2000;7:187–192.
32 Regula J, MacRobert AJ, Gorchein A, Buonaccorsi GA, Thorpe SM, Spencer GM, Hatfield AR, Bown SG: Photosensititsation and photodynamic therapy of oesophageal, duodenal, and colorectal tumours using 5 aminolaevulinic acid induced protoporphyrin IX-a pilot study. Gut 1995;36:67–75.
33 Kelly S, Harris KM, Beery E, Hutton J, Roderick P, Cullingworth J, Gathercole L, Smith MA: A systematic review of the staging performance of endoscopic ultrasound in gastro-oesophageal carcinoma. Gut 2001;49:534–539.
34 Tan WC, Fulljames C, Stone N, Dix AJ, Shepherd N, Roberts DJ, Brown SB, Krasner N, Barr H: Photodynamic therapy using 5-aminolaevulinic acid for oesophageal adenocarcinoma associated with Barrett's metaplasia. J Photochem Photobiol B 1999;53:75–80.
35 Biddlestone LR, Barham CP, Wilkinson SP, Barr H, Shepherd NA: The histopathology of treated Barrett's esophagus: Squamous reepithelialization after acid suppression and laser and photodynamic therapy. Am J Surg Pathol 1998;22:239–245.
36 Barr H: Barrett's esophagus: Treatment with 5-aminolevulinic acid photodynamic therapy. Gastrointest Endosc Clin N Am 2000;10:421–437.
37 Maier A, Tomaselli F, Matzi V, Rehak P, Pinter H, Smolle-Jüttner FM: Does new photosensitizer improve photodynamic therapy in advanced esophageal carcinoma? Lasers in Medical Science 2001;29:328–335.
38 van den Boogert J, van Staveren HJ, de Bruin RW, Eikelaar JH, Siersema PD, van Hillegersberg R: Photodynamic therapy for esophageal lesions: Selectivity depends on wavelength, power, and light dose. Ann Thorac Surg 1999; 68:1763–1769.
39 Overholt BF, Panjehpour M: Barrett's esophagus: Photodynamic therapy for ablation of dysplasia, reduction of specialized mucosa, and treatment of superficial esophageal cancer. Gastrointest Endosc 1995;42:64–70.
40 Okunaka T, Kato H, Conaka C, Yamamoto H, Bonaminio A, Eckhauser ML: Photodynamic therapy of esophageal carcinoma. Surg Endosc 1990;4:150–153.
41 Savary JF, Monnier P, Fontolliet C, Mizeret J, Wagnieres G, Braichotte D, van den Bergh H: Photodynamic therapy for early squamous cell carcinomas of the esophagus, bronchi, and mouth with m-tetra (hydroxyphenyl) chlorin. Arch Otolaryngol Head Neck Surg 1997;123: 162–168.
42 Laukka MA, Wang KK: Initial results using low-dose photodynamic therapy in the treatment of Barrett's esophagus. Gastrointest Endosc 1995;42:59–63.
43 Corti L, Skarlatos J, Boso C, Cardin F, Kosma L, Koukourakis MI, Giatromanolaki A, Norberto L, Shaffer M, Beroukas K: Outcome of patients receiving photodynamic therapy for early esophageal cancer. Int J Radiat Oncol Biol Phys 2000;47:419–424.
44 Panjehpour M, Overholt BF, Haydek JM, Lee SG: Results of photodynamic therapy for ablation of dysplasia and early cancer in Barrett's esophagus and effect of oral steroids on stricture formation. Am J Gastroenterol 2000;95: 2177–2184.
45 Maier A, Tomaselli F, Matzi V, Rehak P, Pinter H, Smolle-Jüttner FM: Photosensitization with hematoporphyrin derivative compared to 5-aminolaevulinic acid for photodynamic therapy of esophageal carcinoma. Ann Thorac Surg 2001;72:1136–1140.
46 Reid BJ: Barrett's esophagus and esophageal adenocarcinoma. Gastroenterol Clin North Am 1991;20:817–834.
47 Stein HJ, Siewert JR: Barrett's esophagus: Pathogenesis, epidemiology, functional abnormalities, malignant degeneration, and surgical management. Dysphagia 1993;8:276–288.
48 Streitz JM Jr, Ellis H Jr: Barrett's esophagus; in Shields TW (ed): General thoracic surgery, ed 4. Baltimore, Williams & Wilkins, 1994, pp 1612–1621.
49 Spechler SJ: Barrett's esophagus. Semin Oncol 1994;21:431–437.
50 Kelsen D, Lauffer I, Leichman L, Orringer MB, Rich TA, Scherl E: Alarming trends in esophageal cancer. Patient Care 1992;October 15:72–122.
51 Provenzale D, Wong JB: Barrett's esophagus and high-grade dysplasia: Immediate esophagectomy versus watchful waiting (abstract). 60th Annual Meeting of the American College of Gastroenterology, 1995.
52 Schnell TG, Sontag SJ, Chejfec G, Aranha G, Metz A, O'Connell S, Seidel UJ, Sonnenberg A: Long-term nonsurgical management of Barrett's esophagus with high-grade dysplasia. Gastroenterology 2001;120:1607–1619.

53 Buttar NS, Wang KK, Sebo TJ, Riehle DM, Krishnadath KK, Lutzke LS, Anderson MA, Petterson TM, Burgart LJ: Extent of high-grade dysplasia in Barrett's esophagus correlated with risk of adenocarcinoma. Gastroenterology 2001;120:1630–1639.
54 Pera M, Cameron AJ, Trastek VF, Carpenter HA, Zinsmeister AR: Increasing incidence of adenocarcinoma of the esophagus and esophagogastric junction. Gastroenterology 1993;104: 510–513.
55 Levine DS, Haggitt RC, Blount PL, Rabinovitch PS, Rusch VW, Reid BJ: An endoscopic biopsy protocol can differentiate high-grade dysplasia from early adenocarcinoma in Barrett's esophagus. Gastroenterology 1993;105: 40–50.
56 Reid BJ, Weinstein WM, Lewin KJ, Haggitt RC, VanDeventer G, DenBesten L, Rubin CE: Endoscopic biopsy can detect high-grade dysplasia or early adenocarcinoma in Barrett's esophagus without grossly recognizable neoplastic lesions. Gastroenterology 1988;94:81–90.
57 Schnell T, Sontag SJ, Chejrec G, et al: High grade dysplasia is not an indication for surgery in patients with Barrett's esophagus (abstract). Gastroenterology 1996;110:A590.
58 Hampton JA, Selman SH: Mechanisms of cell killing in photodynamic therapy using a novel in vivo drug/in vitro light culture system. Photochem Photobiol 1992;56:235–243.
59 Evensen JF, Moan J: Photodynamic action and chromosomal damage: A comparison of haematoporphyrin derivative (HpD) and light with X-irradiation. Br J Cancer 1982;45:456–465.
60 Palley SL, Sampliner RE, Garewal HS: Management of high-grade dysplasia in Barrett's esophagus. J Clin Gastroenterol 1989;11:369–372.
61 Levine DS, Haggitt RC, Irvine S, et al: Natural history of high grade dysplasia in Barrett's esophagus (abstract). Gastroenterology 1996; 110:A550.
62 Montgomery E, Bronner MP, Goldblum JR, Greenson JK, Haber MM, Hart J, Lamps LW, Lauwers GY, Lazenby AJ, Lewin DN, Robert ME, Toledano AY, Shyr Y, Washington K: Reproducibility of the diagnosis of dysplasia in Barrett esophagus: A reaffirmation. Hum Pathol 2001;32:368–378.
63 Gore S, Healey CJ, Sutton R, Eyre-Brook IA, Gear MW, Shepherd NA, Wilkinson SP: Regression of columnar lined (Barrett's) oesophagus with continuous omeprazole therapy. Aliment Pharmacol Ther 1993;7:623–628.
64 Weinstein WM, Lieberman DA, Lewin KJ, et al: Omeprazole-induced regression of Barrett's esophagus: A 2-year randomized controlled double blind trial (abstract). Gastroenterology 1996;110:A294.
65 Gomes MN: Esophageal cancer: Surgical approach; in Ahlgren JD, MacDonald JS (eds): Gastrointestinal Oncology. Philadelphia, Lippincott, 1992, pp 89–121.
66 Levine DS, Haggitt RC, Rabinovich E, et al: Complete regression of high grade dysplasia, DNA content abnormalities, and Barrett's esophagus (abstract). Gastroenterology 1995; 108:A496.
67 Samliner RE, Hixson LJ, Fennerty MB, Garewal HS: Regression of Barrett's esophagus by laser ablation in an acid environment. Dig Dis Sci 1993;38:365–368.
68 Sampliner RE, Fennerty B, Garewal HS: Reversal of Barrett's esophagus with acid suppression and multipolar electrocoagulation: Preliminary results. Gastrointest Endosc 1996;44: 532–535.
69 Jones R, Barham CP, Hardwick R, et al: Regression of columnar-lined esophagus following KTP laser ablation with acid suppression (abstract). Gastroenterology 1996;110:A537.
70 Barham CP, Jones RL, Biddlestone LR, Hardwick RH, Shepherd NA, Barr H: Photothermal laser ablation of Barrett's oesophagus: Endoscopic and histological evidence of squamous re-epithelialisation. Gut 1997;41:281–284.
71 Byrne JP, Armstrong GR: Endoscopic argon beam plasma coagulation in the restoration of squamous lining in Barrett's esophagus. Endoscopy 1997;29:E33.
72 Wang KK, Sampliner RE: Mucosal ablation therapy of Barrett esophagus. Mayo Clin Proc 2001;76:433–437.
73 Ackroyd R, Brown N, Vernon D, Roberts D, Stephenson T, Marcus S, Stoddard C, Reed M: 5-Aminolevulinic acid photosensitization of dysplastic Barrett's esophagus: A pharmacokinetic study. Photochem Photobiol 1999;70: 656–662.
74 van den Boogert J, Houtsmuller AB, de Rooij FW, de Bruin RW, Siersema PD, van Hillegersberg R: Kinetics, localization, and mechanism of 5-aminolevulinic acid-induced porphyrin accumulation in normal and Barrett's-like rat esophagus. Lasers Surg Med 1999;24:3–13.
75 Gossner L, Sroka R, Hahn EG, Ell C: Photodynamic therapy: Successful destruction of gastrointestinal cancer after oral administration of aminolevulinic acid. Gastrointest Endosc 1995;41:55–58.
76 Barr H, Shepherd NA, Dix A, Roberts DJ, Tan WC, Krasner N: Eradication of high-grade dysplasia in columnar-lined (Barrett's) oesophagus by photodynamic therapy with endogenously generated protoporphyrin IX. Lancet 1996; 348:584–585.
77 Ackroyd R, Brown NJ, Davis MF, Stephenson TJ, Marcus SL, Stoddard CJ, Johnson AG, Reed MW: Photodynamic therapy for dysplastic Barrett's oesophagus: A prospective, double blind, randomised, placebo controlled trial. Gut 2000;47:612–617.
78 Kelty C, Ackroyd R: Re-epithelialisation of Barrett's oesophagus. Gut 2001;48:580.
79 Kelty C, Ackroyd R: Re-epithelialisation of Barrett's oesophagus. Gut 2000;47:741.
80 van Laethem JL, Peny MO, Salmon I, Cremer M, Deviere J: Intramucosal adenocarcinoma arising under squamous re-epithelialisation of Barrett's oesophagus. Gut 2000;46:574–577.
81 Krishnadath KK, Wang KK, Taniguchi K, Sebo TJ, Buttar NS, Anderson MA, Lutzke LS, Liu W: Persistent genetic abnormalities in Barrett's esophagus after photodynamic therapy. Gastroenterology 2000;119:624–630.
82 Overholt BF: Results of photodynamic therapy in Barrett's esophagus: A review. Can J Gastroenterol 1999;13:393–396.
83 Messmann H, Mlkvy P, Buonaccorsi G, Davies CL, MacRobert AJ, Bown SG: Enhancement of photodynamic therapy with 5-aminolaevulinic acid-induced porphyrin photosensitisation in normal rat colon by threshold and light fractionation studies. Br J Cancer 1995;72:589–594.
84 Wang KK, Wong Kee Song LM, Nourbakhsh A, Laukka MA, Gutta K, Geller A, Balm R: Controlled trial of low dose photodynamic therapy for Barrett's esophagus (abstract). Gastroenterology 1997;112:A676.
85 Wang KK, Wong Kee Song LM, Nourbakhsh A, Balm R: Can consistent tissue necrosis be achieved during photodynamic therapy for high grade dysplasia or cancer within Barrett's esophagus? (abstract). Gastroenterology 1997; 112:A676.
86 Wang KK, Gutta K, Laukka MA, Alexander GL: A prospective randomized trial of low dose photodynamic therapy in the treatment of Barrett's esophagus (abstract). 5th International Photodynamic Association Biennial Meeting, 1994, p 123.
87 Overholt BF, Panjehpour M: Photodynamic therapy for Barrett's esophagus. Gastrointest Endosc Clin N Am 1997;7:207–220.
88 Beejay U, Ribeiro A, Hourigan L, DeLaMora G, Sanda GCM, Haber GB, Kandel GP, Kortan P, Marcon NE: Photodynamic therapy of high grade dysplasia with intramucosal carcinoma in Barrett's esophagus – 30 months follow-up (abstract). Gastrointest Endosc 2001; 53:AB144.
89 Etienne J, Bourg-Heckley G, Dorme N, Raimbert P, Flejou J-F, Guillemin F: Green light Foscan photodynamic therapy (PDT) on 25 esophageal intramucosal cancers (IMC); in Columbia UoB (ed): International Photodynamic Association 8th World Congress on Photodynamic Medicine. Vancouver, 2001, p 88.
90 Gossner L, May A, Sroka R, Stolte M, Hahn EG, Ell C: Photodynamic destruction of high grade dysplasia and early carcinoma of the esophagus after the oral administration of 5-aminolevulinic acid. Cancer 1999;86:1921–1928.
91 Gossner L, May A, Pech O, Rabenstein T, Schneider HT, Hahn EG, Stolte M, Ell C: Photodynamic therapy of Barrett's esophagus with dysplasia or early cancer (abstract). Gastroenterology 1999;116:A413.
92 Ackroyd R, Brown NJ, Davis MF, Stpehenson TJ, Stoddard CJ, Reed MWR: Anminolaevulinic acid-induced photodynamic therapy in the treatment of dysplastic Barrett's oesophagus and adenocarcinoma. Lasers in Medical Science 1999;14:278–285.

93 Grosjean P, Savary J-F, Wagnieres G, Mizeret J, Woodtl A, Theumann J-F, Fontolliet C, Van den Bergh H, Monnier P: Tetra(m-hydroxy-phenyl)chlorin clinical photodynamic therapy of early bronchial and oesophageal cancers. Lasers in Medical Science 1996;11:227–235.
94 Hayata Y, Kato H, Furuse K, Kunsunoki Y, Suzuki S, Mimura S: Photodynamic therapy of 168 early stage cancers of the lung and oesophagus: A Japanese multi-centre study. Lasers in Medical Science 1996;11:255–259.
95 Messmann H, Szeimies RM, Baumler W, Knuchel R, Zirngibl H, Scholmerich J, Holstege A: Enhanced effectiveness of photodynamic therapy with laser light fractionation in patients with esophageal cancer. Endoscopy 1997;29:275–280.
96 McCaughan JS Jr, Ellison EC, Guy JT, Hicks WJ, Jones JJ, Laufman LR, May E, Nims TA, Spiridonidis CH, Williams TE: Photodynamic therapy for esophageal malignancy: A prospective twelve-year study. Ann Thorac Surg 1996;62:1005–1009.
97 Calzavara F, Tomio L, Corti L, Zorat PL, Barone I, Peracchia A, Norberto L, D'Arcais RF, Berti F: Oesophageal cancer treated by photodynamic therapy alone or followed by radiation therapy. J Photochem Photobiol B 1990;6:167–174.
98 Hayata Y, Kato H, Konaka C, Okitsu H, Suga S, Sayami P: [Laser endoscopy in photodynamic therapy]. Chirurg 1988;59:81–89.
99 Tajiri H, Daikuzono N, Joffe SN, Oguro Y: Photoradiation therapy in early gastrointestinal cancer. Gastrointest Endosc 1987;33:88–90.
100 Fujimaki M, Nakayama K: Endoscopic laser treatment of superficial esophageal cancer. Semin Surg Oncol 1986;2:248–256.
101 Tian ME, Qui SL, Ji Q: Preliminary results of hematoporphyrin derivative-laser treatment for 13 cases of early esophageal carcinoma. Adv Exp Med Biol 1985;193:21–25.
102 Wang KK: Current status of photodynamic therapy of Barrett's esophagus. Gastrointest Endosc 1999;49:S20–S23.

Review Article

Digestive Diseases

Dig Dis 2002;20:18–22

Prevention of Gastric Cancer by *Helicobacter pylori* Eradication?

Results from Clinical Intervention Studies

Laslo Schandl[a,b] Peter Malfertheiner[a] Matthias P.A. Ebert[a]

[a]Department of Gastroenterology, Hepatology and Infectious Diseases, Otto-von-Guericke-University Magdeburg, Germany and [b]2nd Department of Internal Medicine, Semmelweis University Budapest, Hungary

Key Words
Prevention · Gastric cancer · Screening · Infection · *Helicobacter pylori* eradication

Abstract
The incidence of gastric cancer is decreasing; however, in some parts of the world this malignancy is still the second most common cause of cancer-related deaths and recent epidemiological analysis indicates that approximately 1,000,000 individuals will die from gastric cancer every year. Therefore, finding potent mechanisms of cancer prevention is of great importance, since this disease is commonly diagnosed in advanced stages. This review will provide a short update on the mechanisms of gastric carcinogenesis and will present recent data obtained from first clinical intervention studies aimed at the prevention of gastric cancer by *Helicobacter pylori* eradication.

Introduction

Although the incidence of gastric cancer is decreasing in certain parts of the world, it remains the second most common cause of cancer-related death world-wide. Due to several clinical circumstances the diagnosis is often too late and therapeutic options are limited. However, in recent years our understanding of the pathogenesis of gastric cancer has improved and important aspects of its epidemiology, the identification of various molecular alterations and the role of *H. pylori* have been revealed. *H. pylori* was classified in 1994 as a group I carcinogen and extensive sero-epidemiological studies have linked *H. pylori* infection to an increased risk of developing gastric cancer. It resides under microaerobic conditions in a neutral microenvironment between the superficial epithelium and the mucus of the stomach and possesses several virulence factors and stimulates cytokine production by epithelial cells that lead to the activation of immune and inflammatory cells which lead to the damage of host tissues. Multiple gastrointestinal diseases including gastritis, duodenal and gastric ulcer, gastric carcinoma and gastric MALT-lymphoma are associated with *H. pylori* infection, however, the molecular mechanism of their pathogenesis, the role of the host response upon the infection and the genetic background remain largely unkown. This review will focus on novel aspects of gastric cancer pathogenesis, the role of *H. pylori* on the pathogenesis of gastric cancer, and the various strategies that may be useful for the prevention of gastric cancer.

H. pylori Infection and the Process of Gastric Carcinogenesis

Despite a dramatic reduction in incidence and mortality rates, gastric cancer is still one of the most common malignant neoplasias worldwide. Gastric carcinogenesis

KARGER

Fax + 41 61 306 12 34
E-Mail karger@karger.ch
www.karger.com

0257–2753/02/0201–0018$18.50/0

Accessible online at:
www.karger.com/journals/ddi

Dr. M.P.A. Ebert
Department for Gastroenterology, Hepatology and Infectious Diseases
Otto von Guericke University Magdeburg
Leipzigerstrasse 44, D–39120 Magdeburg (Germany), Tel. +49 391 6713156
Fax +49 391 67190054, E-Mail matthias.ebert@medizin.uni-magdeburg.de

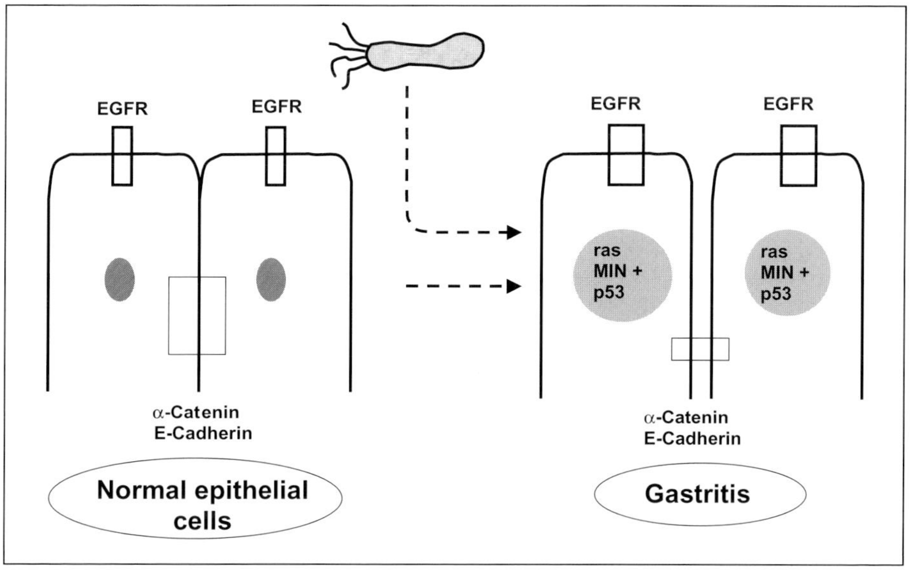

Fig. 1. *H. pylori* infection and alterations of gene expression in the gastric mucosa. In the early phases of gastritis which is induced by *H. pylori* the overexpression of the epidermal growth factor receptor (EGFR), as well as the overexpression of p53 and the presence of microsatellite instability can be identified. The impact of eradication therapy on the regression and reversion of these early molecular changes is still open to debate.

is a complex, multifactorial process, influenced by diet, environment, life style factors, individual susceptibility and *H. pylori* infection [1–3]. A number of epidemiological studies have shown a significant association between *H. pylori* infection of the gastric mucosa and the development of gastric cancer. In the presence of *H. pylori* infection of the gastric mucosa the risk of developing gastric cancer is at least sixfold increased [4–6]. The process of gastric carcinogenesis is believed to be a multi-step process. For the intestinal type of gastric cancer a sequence starting from gastritis to atrophy and intestinal metaplasia, dysplasia and then cancer has been proposed by Correa et al. For diffuse type cancers the histomophological steps leading to gastric cancer are less well defined and largely unkown [7, 8].

Gastric carcinogenesis occurs after a multistep process of genetic and epigenetic alterations in oncogenes, tumor-suppressor genes, cell adhesion molecules, as well as reactivation of the telomerase activity and genetic instability. The activation of oncogenes is one of the hallmarks of molecular gastric carcinogenesis [9]. Numerous studies have demonstrated that *ras* mutations, the aberrant expression of the ras protein product p21, overexpression of *c-erbB2* and other growth factors and growth factor receptors, i.e. hepatocyte growth factor, *K-sam* and *hst-1* are present in the majority of gastric cancers [10]. Interestingly, even the rearrangement of the c-met gene with the tpr gene leading to a TPR-MET fusion hybrid has been reported to occur in gastric cancers [11]. Overexpression of *K-sam* or *hst-1* may be due to gene amplification in a subset of gastric cancers. In about 60% of gastric cancers mutations of the tumor-suppressor gene *p53* have been identified. The alteration of the *APC* gene may also be an early event in gastric cancer pathogenesis [12]. Recent studies indicate that APC controls the degradation of beta-catenin which functions both as an adhesion molecule and transcription factor which induces the expression of cyclin D1. Beta-catenin is frequently overexpressed in gastric cancers, and several groups have reported mutations of this gene in gastric cancers as well. Besides beta-catenin, the expression of other adhesion molecules, such as α-catenin or E-cadherin is frequently altered in gastric cancers [13, 14].

Several studies have tried to identify molecular changes in gastric cancer cells which may directly result from *H. pylori* infection of the gastric mucosa. Interestingly, the great majority of molecular and genetic changes of gastric cancer cells occur independent of *H. pylori* infection [15, 16]. This indicates that the impact of *H. pylori* infection of the gastric mucosa on gastric carcinogenesis seems to be mostly present in the early steps of gastric carcinogenesis or in preneoplastic changes preceding gastric cancer.

H. pylori Infection – Impact on Cell Proliferation, Apoptosis and Cell Adhesion

While the genetic changes in the gastric cancer cells seem to be independent of *H. pylori* infection, *H. pylori* may rather exert its transforming capability through the induction of cellular proliferation and apoptosis in the

Table 1. Clinical intervention studies

Patients	Intervention	Follow-up	Endpoint	Result	Author
n = 122	Hp eradication	12 months	intestinal metaplasia	no change	Hulst 1997
			atrophy	no change	
n = 31	Hp eradication	36 months	mild gastric dysplasia	no change	Farinati 1998
			intestinal metaplasia	worsened	
			atrophy	worsened	
n = 20	Hp eradication	17 months	intestinal metaplasia	no change	Satoh 1998
			atrophy	no change	
n = 251	Hp eradication	6 months	atrophy	no change	Kyzekova 1999
			intestinal metaplasia		
n = 63	Hp eradication	4 years	intestinal metaplasia	no change	Tepes 1999
n = 35	Hp eradication	14 months	adenoma	no change	Gotoda 1999
n = 35	Hp eradication	2 years	intestinal metaplasia	improved	Ciok 1997
n = 53	Hp eradication	12 months	atrophy	improved	Nardone 1999
			intestinal metaplasia	improved	
			cell proliferation	improved	
n = 852	Hp eradication	6-year study	atrophy	improved	Correa 2000
	Beta-carotene, Vit C		intestinal metaplasia		
n = 587	Hp eradication	12 months	intestinal metaplasia	improved	Sung 2000
n = 115	Hp eradication	15 months	atrophy	improved	Ohkusa 2001
			intestinal metaplasia	improved	

histomorphologically normal gastric mucosa. Indeed, in animal models such as the mongolian gerbil *H. pylori* induces active chronic gastritis, ulcers and intestinal metaplasia and in approximately one-third of these cases intestinal-type gastric cancer was induced [17]. In addition, several studies in recent years have shown, that *H. pylori* can induce proliferation of the gastric mucosa. Thus, incubation of AGS gastric epithelial cells with *H. pylori* leads to increased cell proliferation, which was demonstrated by flow-cytometric analysis of Ki-67-positive cells [18]. In addition, *H. pylori* leads to the promotion of apoptosis of gastric epithelial cells in vitro, a process which may be mediated by cytokines, such as interferon-γ or tumor necrosis factor-α [19]. Numerous molecules produced by *H. pylori*, including lipopolysacharide, monochloramide and nitric oxide may directly induce this apoptotic process. Several groups have reported that in the gastric mucosa increased apoptosis and cell proliferation are associated with *H. pylori* infection which correlates with the degree of acute inflammation and the density of *H. pylori* and these latter two factors correlate with each other. Thus, it is hypothesized that *H. pylori* induced apoptosis may play a key role in gastric carcinogenesis by increasing cell proliferation and developing gastric atrophy [20]. In summary, the impact of *H. pylori* on the gastric mucosa includes the induction of cell proliferation, the induction of apoptosis and the reduction of cellular adhesion (fig. 1).

Molecular and Morphological Changes after *H. pylori* Eradication

The preneoplastic lesions leading to gastric cancer are largely undefined. Various studies indicate that atrophy and intestinal metaplasia may present preneoplastic lesions of the stomach [21, 22]. However, recent studies indicate that these histomorphological changes may rather present markers of an increased risk of developing gastric cancer [23, 24]. Thus, intestinal metaplasia and atrophy are frequently cited in the literature as risk indicators of *H. pylori* infection and an increased risk of developing gastric cancer [23, 24]. *H. pylori* gastritis, particularly in the corpus is significantly more frequent in gastric carcinoma patients or individuals with family history of gastric carcinoma [25]. Therefore, the presence of a corpus-predominant gastritis with or without intestinal metaplasia has been proposed to be a risk condition for the development of gastric cancer [26, 27]. Furthermore, in relatives of patients with gastric cancer *H. pylori* infection and the presence of a corpus-dominant gastritis, atrophy and intestinal metaplasia are significantly more frequent as compared to individuals without a family history of gastric cancer [27]. Furthermore, apoptosis and cell proliferation are increased in precancerous lesions such as gastric atrophy, intestinal metaplasia and dysplasia in the presence of *H. pylori* infection [24].

Table 2. Intervention studies and molecular changes

A Intervention studies and molecular changes

Patients	Intervention	Follow-up	Result	Author
n = 53	Hp eradication	12 months	reduction of PCNA expression; loss of p53 and c-myc expression	Nardone 1999
n = 31	Hp eradication	4 weeks	reduced TUNEL-labeling index; reduced Ki67 expression	Hoshi 1999
n = 17	Hp eradication	12 months	COX-2 expression reduced	Sung 2000

B Intervention studies in animal models

Animal model	Treatment	Follow-up	Result	Author
Mongolian gerbils	Hp inoculation and eradication	50 weeks	Reduced cases of gastric cancers following eradication	Shimizu 2000

Prevention of gastric cancer by *H. pylori* eradication presents an interesting option. In order to evaluate different intervention stategies the endpoints of these interventions need to be clearly defined. While the prevention of cancer is the primary target, however, these studies using cancer prevention as the primary target need a long follow-up. Therefore, the definition of preneoplastic lesions of the stomach is of high interest. Based on previous considerations, several groups have used cell proliferation, atrophy and intestinal metaplasia as endpoints for their intervention studies. Interestingly, up to date almost as many positive as negative studies have been published (tables 1, 2). The critical point seems to be the follow-up which ranges from 4 weeks to 4 years. In addition, the design of the study varies greatly and placebo-controlled prospective studies are very rare. Most studies rely on the retrospective analysis of biopsies taken after eradication. Several groups have reported that gastric cell proliferation is significantly higher in patients with *H. pylori* infection than in normal controls, and eradication of the infection leads to a reduction in cell proliferation. [21, 22, 28]. In contrast, reversibility of intestinal metaplasia after eradication is still under discussion. In a study by Sakaki et al. [29] the regression of intestinal metaplasia even 2 years after successful *H. pylori* eradication was not observed. However, Nardone et al. reported the restoration of DNA aneuploidy, and p53 and c-myc overexpression one year after eradication of *H. pylori*, whereas these marker remained unchanged in patients in whom *H. pylori* persisted [28]. A positive finding in terms of successful regression of histomorphological changes following *H. pylori* eradication, however, should be considered only with great caution. Nonetheless, intervention studies in mongolian gerbils after inoculation of *Helicobacter* have found a reduced number of gastric cancer (table 3). Furthermore, identifying molecular markers of individuals who might benefit from an erdication therapy are still underway (table 2). Inasmuch as human studies using gastric cancer prevention as the primary endpoint are still missing the value of *Helicobacter* eradication as a means for the prevention of gastric cancer still remains a possible option and studies using molecular changes might be useful to identify individuals which would benefit from *H. pylori* eradication as a cancer preventive strategy.

Conclusion

Several epidemiological, pathophysiological and histomorphological studies have linked *H. pylori* to the development of gastric cancer. However, the genetic and molecular mechanisms underlying its pathogenesis remain largely unkown. Recent studies investigating premalignant lesions of gastric cancer and their potential to revert after eradication therapy have led to considerable discussion whether eradication therapy should be offered to individuals for the prevention of gastric cancer. In fact, the etiology of gastric cancer underlies several factors, including hereditary risk, low socio-economic status, increased uptake of nitrates, decreased intake of vitamines and smoking, as well as *H. pylori* infection [3]. Interestingly, *H. pylori* infection is the easiest candidate for treatment and therefore, presents one of the few options that can be controlled in order to reduce the risk of developing gastric cancer. To date and based on latest results from Japan *H. pylori* is the essential trigger for gastric carcinogenesis with up to 100% of gastric cancers attributed to this infection [30]. Furthermore, other large studies from the recent years clearly demonstrate that *H. pylori* is associated with gastric carcinogenesis, it leads to gastric cancer in the animal model of mongolian gerbils, its presence in risk groups is associated with an increased frequency of premalignant lesions and conditions and, finally, several studies have demonstrated the restoration and reversion of morphological and molecular changes after eradication therapy. Thus, several arguments favour the eradication therapy as a means to prevent gastric cancer in infected individuals. However, since not all patients with *H. pylori* infection will develop gastric cancer, it seems to be advisable to limit the preventive eradication therapy to individuals with an increased risk of developing gastric cancer, i.e. first-degree relatives, patients with early gastric cancer after resection of the tumor, and probably individuals with potential preneoplastic lesions of the stomach.

Acknowledgements

L. Schandl was supported by the DAAD. M.P.A. Ebert is supported by the DAAD, DFG and the Land Sachsen-Anhalt.

References

1 Ekstrom AM, Hansson LE, Signorello LB, Lindgren A, Bergstrom R, Nyren O: Decreasing incidence of both major histologic subtypes of gastric adenocarcinoma – a population-based study in Sweden. Br J Cancer 2000;83: 392–396.

2 Huang JQ, Hunt RH: Helicobacter pylori and gastric cancer – the clinician's point of view. Aliment Pharmacol Ther 2000;14:48–54.

3 Sipponen P, Marshall BJ: Gastritis and gastric cancer. Western countries. Gastroenterol Clin North Am 2000;29:579–592.

4 Graham DY: Helicobacter pylori infection is the primary cause of gastric cancer. J Gastroenterol 2000;35:90–97.

5 Haruma K, Komoto K, Kamada T, Ito M, Kitadai Y, Yoshihara M, Sumii K, Kajiyama G: Helicobacter pylori infection is a major risk factor for gastric carcinoma in young patients. Scand J Gastroenterol 2000;35:255–259.

6 Limburg PJ, Qiao YL, Mark SD, Wang GQ, Perez-Perez GI, Blaser MJ, Wu YP, Zou XN, Dong ZW, Taylor PR, Dawsey SM: Helicobacter pylori seropositivity and subsite-specific gastric cancer risk in Linxian, China. J Natl Cancer Inst 2001;93:226–233.

7 Correa P: Human gastric carcinogenesis: a multistep and multifactorial process – first American Cancer Society Award Lecture on cancer epidemiology and prevention. Cancer Res 1992;52:6735–6740.

8 Lauren, P: The two histological main types of gastric carcinoma: diffuse and so-called intestinal type carcinoma. Acta Pathol Microbiol Scand 1955;64:31–49.

9 Tahara E, Semba S, Tahara H: Molecular biological observations in gastric cancer. Semin Oncol 1996;23:307–315.

10 Park JB, Rhim JS, Park SC, Kimm SW, Kraus MH: Amplification, overexpression and rearrangement of the c-erbB2 protooncogene in primary human stomach carcinomas. Cancer Res 1989;49:6605–6609.

11 Yu J, Ebert M, Miehlke S, Breidert T, Pich U, Starzynska T, Bayerdörffer E, Malfertheiner P: Detection of the TPR-MET rearrangement in patients with gastric cancer and relatives. Gastroenterology 1999;116:A397.

12 Hsieh LL, Huang YC: Loss of heterozygosity of APC/MCC gene in differentiated and undifferentiated gastric carcinoma in Taiwan. Cancer Lett 1995;96:169–174.

13 Jawhari A, Jordan S, Poole S, Browne P, Pignatelli M, Farthing MJG: Abnormal immunoreactivity of the E-cadherin-catenin complex in gastric carcinoma: relationship with patient survival. Gastroenterology 1997;112:46–54.

14 Becker KF, Atkinson MJ, Reich U, Becker I, Nekarda H, Siewert JR, Hofler H: E-cadherin gene mutations provide clues to diffuse type gastric carcinomas. Cancer Res 1994;54:3845–3852.

15 Ebert MPA, Yu J, Sung JJ, Malfertheiner P: Molecular alterations in gastric cancer: the role of H. pylori. Eur J Gastro Hepatol 2000;12: 795–798.

16 Wu MS, Shun CT, Wang HP, Sheu JC, Lee WJ, Wang TH, Lin JT: Genetic alterations in gastric cancer: relation to histological subtypes, tumor stage, and Helicobacter pylori infection. Gastroenterology 1997;112:1457–1465.

17 Watanabe T, Tada M, Nagai H, Sasaki S, Nakao M: Helicobacter pylori infection induces gastric cancer in mongolian gerbils. Gastroenterology 1998;115:642–648.

18 Fan XG, Kelleher D, Fan XJ, Xia HX, Keeling PWN: Helicobacter pylori increases proliferation of gastric epithelial cells. Gut 1996;38:19–22.

19 Wagner S, Beil W, Westermann J, Logan RPH, Bock CT, Trautwein C, Bleck JS, Manns MP: Regulation of gastric epithelial cell growth by Helicobacter pylori: evidence for a major role of apoptosis. Gastroenterology 1997;113: 1836–1847.

20 Goldstone AR, Quirke P, Dixon MF: Helicobacter pylori infection and gastric cancer. J Pathol 1996;179:129–137.

21 Jang TJ, Kim JR: Proliferation and apoptosis in gastric antral epithelial cells of patients infected with Helicobacter pylori. J Gastroenterol 2000;35:265–271.

22 Takagi A, Watanabe S, Igarashi M, Koike J, Hasumi K, Deguchi R, Koga Y, Miwa T: The effect of Helicobacter pylori on cell proliferation and apoptosis in gastric epithelial cell lines. Aliment Pharmacol Ther 2000;14:188–192.

23 Dixon MF: Atrophy, metaplasia, and dysplasia – a risk for gastric cancer: are they reversible? in Hunt RH, Tytgat GNJ (eds): Helicobacter pylori; Basic Mechanisms to Clinical Cure 1998. Dordrecht, Kluwer Academic Publishers, 1998, pp 336–353.

24 Malfertheiner P: Helicobacter pylori – von der Grundlage zur Therapie. Stuttgart, Thieme, 2000.

25 Miehlke S, Hackelsberger A, Meining A, von Arnim U, Müller P, Ochsenkühn T, Lehn N, Malfertheiner P, Stolte M, Bayerdörffer E: Histological diagnosis of Helicobacter pylori gastritis is predictive of a high risk of gastric carcinoma. Int J Cancer 1997;73:837–839.

26 Meining A, Bayerdörffer E, Müller P, Miehlke S, Lehn N, Hölzel D, Hatz R, Stolte M: Gastric carcinoma risk index in patients infected with Helicobacter pylori. Virchows Arch 1998;432: 311–314.

27 El-Omar EM, Ojen K, Murray LS, El-Nujumi A, Wirz A, Gillen D: Increased prevalence of precancerous changes in relatives of gastric cancer patients. Gastroenterology 2000;118: 22–30

28 Nardone G, Staibano S, Rocco A, Mezza E, D'Armiento FP, Insabato L, Coppola A, Salvatore G, Lucariello A, Figura N, De Rosa G, Budillon G: Effect of Helicobacter pylori infection and its eradication on cell proliferation, DNA status, and oncogene expression in patients with chronic gastritis. Gut 1999;44:789–799.

29 Sakaki N, Kozawa H: Intestinal metaplasia and *Helicobacter pylori* infection, their relationship and effects of eradication therapy. Nippon Rinsho 2001;59:361–366.

30 Uemura N, Okamoto S, Yamamoto S, Matsumura N, Yamaguchi S, Yamakido M, Taniyama K, Sasaki N, Schlemper RJ: Helicobacter pylori infection and the development of gastric cancer. N Engl J Med 2001;345:784–789.

Review Article

Digestive Diseases

Dig Dis 2002;20:23–31

E-Cadherin Mutations and Hereditary Gastric Cancer: Prevention by Resection?

R.C. Fitzgerald C. Caldas

Hutchison/MRC Research Centre, Cambridge, UK

Key Words

E-cadherin · Gastric cancer · Prevention

Abstract

Background: A small percentage of gastric cancers (1–3%) arise as a result of clearly identified inherited gastric cancer predisposition syndromes. Recently, linkage analysis has implicated E-cadherin (CDH1) mutations in a subset of dominantly inherited gastric cancers termed hereditary diffuse gastric cancer (HDGC). Heterozygotes with the CDH1 mutation have a 70–80% chance of developing gastric cancer and once patients have invasive, symptomatic disease there is a high associated morbidity and mortality. As a result prophylactic gastrectomy has been advocated for affected family members identified by genetic screening. There are many issues to be considered in order to determine whether prophylactic gastrectomy is the optimal management strategy for these patients. ***Methods:*** A MEDLINE literature search was performed and combined with our own experience in order to identify relevant background information on hereditary gastric cancer. In particular we extracted information about prophylactic gastrectomy in HDGC patients. ***Results:*** Once the decision has been undertaken to perform genetic testing, the therapeutic options are either endoscopic screening with the aim of identifying an early, curable lesion or prophylactic surgery. Two groups have published their data on prophylactically resected stomachs in asymptomatic patients from affected families. In these series all of the post-gastrectomy specimens had microscopic evidence of diffuse gastric cancer confined within the mucosal layer. These early cancers had not been identified by endoscopic surveillance. Technical issues surrounding the age at which to operate, the best operation to reduce the risk of postoperative complications and the risk of other cancers developing in other organs in these patients are still controversial. Long-term follow-up studies in specialist centres are required to resolve these issues. ***Conclusions:*** From the limited experience so far the estimated risk reduction of gastric cancer by gastrectomy is significant.

Introduction

Gastric cancer is the second largest cancer burden worldwide [1]. Although there has been a decreasing incidence in gastric cancer globally, it remains a major public health concern because of the low survival rates (10% at

KARGER

Fax + 41 61 306 12 34
E-Mail karger@karger.ch
www.karger.com

0257–2753/02/0201–0023$18.50/0

Accessible online at:
www.karger.com/journals/ddi

Dr. Rebecca Fitzgerald
Hutchison/MRC Research Centre
Hills Road
Cambridge, CB2 2XZ (UK)
Tel. +44 1223 763287, Fax +44 1223 763296, E-Mail rcf@hutchison-mrc.cam.ac.uk

Table 1. Inherited gastric cancer predisposition syndromes

Disorder	Manifestations	Inheritance	Gene(s) detected
Familial adenomatous polyposis (FAP)	Multiple GI polyps, especially colonic	autosomal dominant	APC
Hereditary non-polyposis colon cancer (HNPCC) type b or Lynch II	familial colorectal cancer, members prone to cancer of female genital tract and other sites	autosomal dominant	mismatch repair genes hMSH2 hMLH7 hPMS1 hPMS2
Peutz-Jeghers syndrome	hamartomatous polyps throughout gut + orocutaneous melanin spots lifetime prevalence small bowel adenoma 2.4%	autosomal dominant variable and incomplete penetrance	not known
Cowden's syndrome	multiple hamartomas and multiple mucocutaneous manifestations and increased risk of malignancy 40% have GI lesions, mainly colonic	autosomal dominant	not known
Li-Fraumeni syndrome	may develop a variety of tumours including breast, sarcomas, leukaemia, brain, GI tract rarely affected	autosomal dominant	p53

5 years) [2, 3]. The poor prognosis of gastric cancer can largely be attributed to late presentation and diagnosis. In contrast to the West, Japan has introduced systematic mass screening programmes which have led to increased detection rates of gastric cancers confined to the mucosa or submucosa (so called early gastric cancers) [4]. Unlike the low survival rates usually associated with gastric cancer, patients with early gastric cancers have 5-year survival rates in excess of 90% independent of their histological subtype. Hence, this would suggest that if all gastric cancers could be detected early then this would enable improved prognosis. Aside from mass screening programmes which have large cost implications and may be impractical, another approach would be to try to identify those individuals at high risk for developing gastric cancer.

The major risk factor for intestinal gastric cancer identified so far is *Helicobacter pylori* infection [5–7]. However, whether *H. pylori* eradication is an effective cancer prevention measure has not been proven [6]. In contrast to these sporadic occurrences of gastric cancer, a small percentage of gastric cancers (1–3%) arise as a result of clearly identified inherited gastric cancer predisposition syndromes [8–11] (table 1). The existence of a familial form of gastric cancer has been known about since the 1800s, when multiple cases of gastric cancer were noted in the Bonaparte family [12].

Gastric cancers can be classified in terms of their anatomical site and histopathological subtype. The two major histopathological subtypes are the intestinal type and the diffuse or linitis plastica type. The diffuse types are commoner in endemic areas, tend to have a poorer prognosis and their aetiopathology is less well understood. A subset of these diffuse type gastric cancers are hereditary and recently linkage analysis has implicated E-cadherin (CDH1) mutations in an estimated 25% of them [13]. This subset of gastric cancer has been termed hereditary diffuse gastric cancer (HDGC).

It is perhaps not surprising that E-cadherin has been implicated in HDGC since in 1994 Becker et al. identified somatic E-cadherin mutations in specimens of diffuse gastric cancer [14]. Since then CDH1 mutations have been found in 40–83% sporadic diffuse cancers but not in intestinal-type gastric cancers [15–17]. The diffuse phenotype probably occurs as a result of aberrant cell-cell adhesion secondary to abnormal E-cadherin expression. A causal role for E-cadherin has been demonstrated in the transition from adenoma to carcinoma in a mouse model of pancreatic tumour progression [18] and silencing of E-cadherin has been described in human carcinomas [19]. So far, there has only been one report of an E-cadherin germline mutation in an apparently sporadic gastric cancer [20].

As a result of the identification of the genetic mutation responsible for HDGC there are far reaching clinical sequelae. First, there is the question of identifying asymptomatic individuals from affected families and providing genetic testing to see if they harbour a CDH1 mutation. Second, once an affected individual is identified there is the opportunity to try to prevent invasive gastric cancer from developing. The current options are regular endoscopic surveillance or else the seemingly radical option of a prophylactic gastrectomy. After a brief review of the clinical and molecular characteristics of this disease, the ramifications of prophylactic gastrectomy are discussed in detail.

Characteristics of HDGC

As noted already, the histopathology of HDGC is uniformly of the diffuse linitis plastica type of cancer although a minority of tumours may also have a glandular/intestinal component [21]. To determine whether the HDGCs have any distinctive pathological features among all diffuse carcinomas will require a controlled and blinded analysis of a larger number of such specimens.

The age of onset is typically much younger than sporadic gastric cancers. There is an average age of 38 years compared with sporadic cancer which tends to occur in 60–70 year olds. The youngest cases of HDGC reported have been in persons under 18 years of age.

In order to be considered for a diagnosis of HDGC the following criteria have to be met [22]: (1) two or more documented cases of diffuse gastric cancer in first or second degree relatives, with at least one diagnosed before the age of 50 or (2) three or more cases of documented DGC in 1st/2nd degree relatives, independently of age of onset.

These criteria were set to be over inclusive in order to collect gastric cancer families and to identify other predisposing gene(s). Hence, in a study of Finnish and Japanese gastric cancer families, in which not all of the cases had a diffuse histopathological subtype, no CDH1 mutations were found [23, 24]. Despite the negative Finnish and Japanese data, HDGC families harbouring CDH1 mutations have been identified from varied ethnic backgrounds (Caucasian, Japanese, Korean, African-American), [13, 14, 25, 26]. Therefore, HDGC does not seem to be restricted to one ethnic group but the inclusion/exclusion criteria are likely to be critical in order to identify affected individuals.

Research on these families has also shown that penetrance of the gene is high, with an estimated range of 70–80%; therefore if you carry the abnormal E-cadherin gene you have a 70–80% lifetime risk of developing gastric cancer [27]. This high penetrance is similar to medullary thyroid cancers in MEN2 syndromes and breast cancer in BRCA1 carriers.

The longest follow-up data of patients with HDGC comes from Maori kindred which were first described in 1964. Indeed, it was from this kindred that Guilford et al. first identified the germline mutations of CDH1 in 1998 [13]. In this kindred over 25 family members have died from gastric cancer, with an increased frequency of colorectal cancer in these patients. The age of death from gastric cancer ranges from 14 years and the majority of affected persons die when they are under 40 years of age. Hence, data from these Maori families and from other series suggest that individuals with CDH1 mutations may be predisposed to the development of other cancers (lobular breast, colorectal and prostate) [20, 28, 27]. However, it was felt that the inclusion of other associated cancers into the definition of HDGC was too premature [22].

The working definition for HDGC appears to be fulfilling its aims since recent work has shown that whereas 36.4% of families fulfilling the criteria for HDGC harboured CDH1 mutations, no mutations were found in those kindred not fulfilling the criteria [29].

Locus and Genetic Abnormalities of CDH1

Before discussing the clinical implications of CDH1 mutations with regards to genetic testing and therapeutic strategies, it is important to appreciate the molecular genetics of these tumours since clearly future methods to obviate the need for gastric surgery are preferable.

The analysis of all the reported genetic abnormalities in CDH1 found in HDGC reveals that the majority are inactivating mutations (splice-site, frameshift and nonsense) rather then missense. Furthermore, the CDH1 germline mutations are evenly distributed along the E-cadherin gene, in contrast to the clustering in exons 7–9 observed in sporadic diffuse gastric cancer [30]. These germline mutations affect one allele, leaving a wild-type E-cadherin allele.

CDH1 is a tumour suppressor gene and hence loss or inactivation of the remaining normal allele would be expected to be a required initiating event in susceptible individuals with a germline mutation. The 'second hit' is normally deletion of the whole gene or else silencing of the

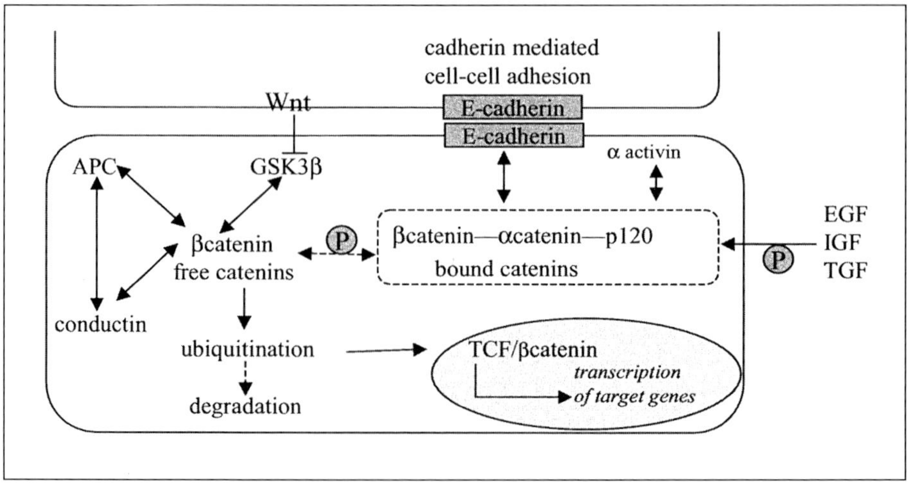

Fig. 1. Simplified schema for the role of cadherins and catenins in signal transduction. Catenins are redistributed between the bound and the 'free' state (cadherin-independent cytoplasmic pool) depending upon their phosphorylation state (shown as encircled P). The phosphorylation state can be influenced by extracellular growth factors (epidermal growth factor EGF, insulin like growth factor IGF and transforming growth factors TGF) and by the Wnt signalling pathway. In the absence of Wnt-1 ligand the levels of β -catenin are kept low due to a high turnover rate by proteolytic degradation. This default route involves phosphorylation and interaction with the tumour suppressor (Adenomatous Polyposis Coli) APC and glycogen synthase kinase 3β (GSK 3β). In cancer mutational alterations, such as inactivating APC, GSKβ mutations or β-catenin mutations, may lead to an increase in the free cytoplasmic pool of catenin and hence via transcriptional activation may promote neoplastic growth.

gene by promoter methylation. Aberrant CDH1 promoter methylation has been demonstrated in three out of six HDGC with negative E-cadherin expression [31]. Reduction of E-cadherin expression by hypermethylation of the CDH1 promoter region is common in a number of non-inherited tumours such as breast, prostate, hepatocellular and thyroid [32, 33, 19] as well as in sporadic diffuse gastric cancer [34]. Interestingly, a demethylating agent, 5-azacytidine, restored E-cadherin expression in a gastric cancer cell line (SNU-1) that tested positive for promoter CDH1 methylation [35]. Hence, it is tempting to consider the potential value of prophylactic treatment of these mutation carriers with demethylating agents such as 5-azadeoxycytidine.

In contrast, some individuals with germline E-cadherin mutations have E-cadherin protein detectable immunohistochemically. Hence it has been suggested that the germline mutations identified have a dominant negative effect similar to forms of N-cadherin in embryonic cell adhesion [36]. Alternatively, it has also been suggested that a 50% reduction in E-cadherin function may be sufficient to promote tumourigenesis.

E-Cadherin Protein Function

E-cadherin is a 120 kDa calcium-dependent adhesion molecule that is a member of the cadherin family of proteins, a class of cell surface proteins that establish intercellular connections through homophilic interactions and maintain epithelial tissue polarity and structural integrity. The E-cadherin gene coding sequence gives rise to a 27 amino acid signal peptide (exons 1–2), a 154 amino acid precursor peptide (exons 2–4) and a 728 amino acid mature protein [30]. This mature protein consists of 3 major domains, a large extracellular domain (exons 4–13) and smaller transmembrane domains (exons 13–14) and cytoplasmic domains (exons 14–16). The extracellular portion mediates homophilic interactions, whereas its intracellular part provides a link to the actin cytoskeleton through an association with the catenins (α, β, δ). One of these, β-catenin, is not only involved in cell adhesion but also in signal transduction (fig. 1).

The mechanism by which these E-cadherin mutations actually lead to cancer is probably complex. It is likely that disrupted cell-cell adhesion could play a role in the initiation of cell proliferation by allowing escape from growth control signals. Furthermore, the cytoplasmic domain of E-cadherin may modulate the Wnt signalling pathway by inhibiting the availability of free cytoplasmic β catenin, in a manner complimentary to the product of the colorectal tumour suppressor APC (fig. 1).

Underexpression of E-cadherin protein is a prognostic marker of poor clinical outcome in many tumour types [37]. Specifically, there is overwhelming evidence that loss of E-cadherin function is associated with invasiveness, lymph node metastasis, distant metastasis and other poor prognostic factors [1, 38–40]. Furthermore, restored E-cadherin expression in tumour models can suppress invasiveness of epithelial tumour cells [41, 42]. Recently, Perl et al. used a transgenic mouse model of pancreatic beta cell tumourigenesis to demonstrate that abrogation of E-cadherin mediated cell adhesion induces tumour invasion and metastasis [18]. However, since loss of membranous staining appears to be a late event in tumourigenesis this would be unlikely to be clinically useful for identifying early gastric cancers.

Genetic Testing and Counselling for Families at Risk for HDGC

The first step for reducing the incidence of HDGC is to identify asymptomatic persons at risk and to offer genetic testing. It is recognised that E-cadherin testing involves uncertainty about clinical management, disease outcome and imposes a psychosocial burden on the family member [22]. However, in light of the highly lethal nature of HDGC which is autosomal dominant with a high degree of penetrance for heterozygotes, withholding this information may do more harm than good. Deliberate and thoughtful counselling and consultation with family members, external counsellors and advisers is an essential component of genetic testing. Experience has also found that counselling with other patients who have had a gastrectomy may be helpful. It has been suggested that the counselling framework should be the same as that for other family cancer syndromes with several separate phases. Firstly, diagnostic testing for E-cadherin mutations in the germline should be conducted on a sample from an affected subject (a family member with gastric cancer). The samples should be in the form of whole blood, banked DNA or paraffin tissue. If paraffin samples are the only available option due to death of the affected member then paraffin blocks on two separate cases should be analysed to avoid artefactual results. The results of the genetic testing should then be confirmed by an independent clinical (as opposed to a research) laboratory.

In the second phase, if the symptomatic family member is positive for CDH1 mutations then asymptomatic family members are tested. Each family member tested must be given counselling both before and after the testing is performed. This counselling should be provided by a multidisciplinary group of clinicians. The team should review and discuss the natural history of HDGC, the risk for that individual given what is known about the genetics (70% lifetime risk from data so far which is based on small numbers), the possible outcomes of the test and the therapeutic options. The impact on health and life insurability, as well as other psychosocial issues should also be addressed. If an asymptomatic family member wishes to proceed with genetic testing then informed consent must be obtained and submitted with the sample.

If the testing for CDH1 mutations is negative then it should be explained to the subject that their risk of developing gastric cancer is the same as for the general population. In this circumstance then no further action is needed. If on the other hand the testing proves positive then this must be confirmed in a separate clinical laboratory. If confirmed then the affected person has to reach a decision about their preferred clinical management.

Age of Testing

The age at which genetic testing (and gastrectomy) should be performed is not yet clear from the current evidence. At least five subjects have been reported to develop this lethal cancer before the age of 18 years [13, 43]. It has therefore been argued that genetic testing should be made available for children in a way similar to that for families affected by multiple endocrine neoplasia (MEN2) and familial adenomatous polyposis (FAP), [22]. However, the implications of the diagnosis are far-reaching in terms of prophylatic gastrectomy and it is the opinion of the authors that genetic screening should be reserved until the patient is able to make informed consent.

Consideration of the age of onset of this disease also raises the possibility that environmental factors may play a role. Although *H. pylori* infection is generally associated with intestinal type gastric cancers, a close association has been observed between diffuse gastric cancer and infection in a younger generation of patients [44, 45]. Interestingly an elevated frequency of cagA producing cytotoxic strains has been documented in New Zealand Polynesians in contrast to New Zealanders of European descent [46]. Epidemiological studies that compare the incidence of early and late onset cancer in HDGC families should provide a powerful approach for the identification of environmental factors which influence the onset of both sporadic and familial gastric cancer.

Risk of Affected Members Developing Other Cancers

Due to the increased incidence of other cancers in individuals with CDH1 mutations it needs to be considered whether it is necessary to provide screening for other cancers (e.g. for breast [43, 40] and colonic cancers [28]). The family data collected by member groups of the International Gastric Cancer Linkage Consortium confirms that women with CDH1 mutations have a significant lifetime risk of breast cancer as well as diffuse gastric cancer [27]. The cumulative risk of breast cancer in these individuals is 39% by aged 80 years. However, the gastric cancer penetrance is much higher, and a mutation carrier is almost 5 times more likely to develop gastric cancer than breast cancer. With regards to colon cancer the combined epidemiological data [47] do not support that E-cadherin alterations predispose to colon cancer in families with gastric and colon cancer. Interestingly, the prevalence of CDH1 mutations among sporadic colon cancer patients was higher in Sweden than that in Finland and Norway [47]. Hence, it is possible that there might be another modifying genetic alteration, more prevalent in Sweden, which increases the risk for colorectal cancer in association with an E-cadherin mutation in the Swedish population.

However, the possibility cannot be excluded that the incidence of these other malignancies is coincidental. For example, it is not clear how mutation of an epithelial adhesion molecule would predispose to leukaemia [20]. So although there may be a slightly increased risk of CDH1 mutant carriers developing cancers other than gastric cancers the risk would appear to be small and so far no patients have developed other cancers post-gastrectomy. Hence, at the current time screening for other malignancies, other than possibly breast cancer, is not recommended.

Clinical Management of Affected Persons

The therapeutic options currently available are either endoscopic screening with the aim of identifying an early, curable lesion or prophylactic gastrectomy.

Endoscopic gastric cancer surveillance is unproven because the lesions are submucosal and hence biopsies may not detect the abnormality. Furthermore, the affected area may be localised and so the early cancer may not be detected as a result of sampling error. In an effort to improve the diagnostic yield of surveillance endoscopy, techniques such as chromoendoscopy (methylene blue or indigo carmine dye spraying), endoscopic ultrasound and optical endoscopic methods (such as optical coherence tomography, elastic scattering spectroscopy and autofluorescence) have been evaluated. Many of these techniques are also being evaluated for use in oesophageal cancer surveillance in patients with Barrett's oesophagus in which there are some parallel challenges. In this disease, dysplasia is also extremely heterogeneous and the abnormal areas are frequently not visible macroscopically. However, to date none of these techniques has been proven to improve the diagnostic yield in gastric or for that matter in oesophageal cancer.

The alternative approach to endoscopic surveillance is to perform a prophylactic gastrectomy. It is useful to review the limited worldwide experience of this approach. Two groups [48–50] showed that prophylactically resected stomachs from different families all carried multifocal signet ring cancer. Importantly, surveillance using endoscopy (with chromoendoscopy in some cases) and multiple mucosal biopsies had failed to identify intramucosal carcinoma in all of the cases surveilled. The remarkable fact is that the operations which were considered to be prophylactic turned out to be therapeutic and curative.

Hence from these limited examples, the estimated risk reduction of gastric cancer by gastrectomy is significant. It should be noted that not all families have such high gene penetrance as in the cases reported so far in the literature. It follows that since there is an estimated 70% penetrance, then a universal policy of prophylactic gastrectomy would result in 30% of HDGC mutation carriers receiving an unnecessary operation. For those patients who refuse a prophylactic gastrectomy it would seem sensible to recommend *H. pylori* eradication therapy in order to minimise the risk of other gastric carcinogens.

It is interesting to compare the experience of prophylactic gastrectomy with other prophylactic cancer surgery such as mastectomy performed for individuals with the hereditary breast cancer syndrome secondary to BRCA1 and BRCA2 germline mutations. Prophylactic mastectomy specimens have been shown to harbour occult foci of malignant cells, even in the setting of negative mammograms [51, 52]. Furthermore, prophylactic mastectomy reduces the risk of breast cancer by 90%. However, this reduction in breast cancer has to be offset against the associated negative effects on self-esteem and sexual function. There are similar considerations to be taken into account with regards to gastric cancer.

Technical Considerations of Gastrectomy [50]

Operating on young, fit individuals is a different thing altogether than operating on patients with symptomatic gastric cancer. When a patient has gastric cancer then it is a much more major surgery with a higher associated morbidity and mortality. However, at the current time there is very limited data on the outcome for prophylactic gastrectomy for asymptomatic individuals.

The optimal type of reconstruction is debatable. The options are: (1) Reconstruction via a Roux-en-Y direct limb; (2) use of an interposed jejunal graft to allow oesophago-jejunal-duodenal reconstruction, and construction of a pouch of jejunum just distal to oesophageal anastamosis to provide larger reservoir for food versus direct connection of the isoperistaltic jejunum.

Several groups have studied these issues and although it appears that jejunal interposition between oesophagus and duodenum may have a slight advantage in maintenance of weight, this is at the cost of significantly increased bile reflux and an additional anastamosis which increases the risk of technical complications. Hence, a Roux-en Y is probably preferable [53–55].

It has also been reported that failure to accurately predict the level of the gastro-oesophageal junction has resulted in two patients requiring an additional resection to ensure that all gastric mucosa is removed [50]. As a result of this it has been suggested that an upper GI endoscopy performed on the operating table may be necessary in order to help to identify the squamocolumnar junction. It has also been suggested that frozen sections should be taken at the same time to verify the anatomical limits of the gastric mucosa. Whilst other discussants felt that this was unnecessary, it was agreed that in order to minimise the cancer risk that all gastric tissue must be excised [50].

Post-Operative Complications

The postoperative complications following a gastrectomy have been extensively reviewed previously, and are summarised here in table 2. Clearly, these results need to be tempered for young fit individuals. Long-term follow-up is required in order to assess their ability to return to work and effects on their quality of life [21].

Table 2. Postoperative complications of gastrectomy

	Estimated frequency, %
Short term complications	
30-day mortality	3–6
Leakage rates	8–12
Wound and intra-abdominal complications	5–10
Longer-term metabolic complications	
Postoperative weight loss at 3–6 months	100
10–15% permanent decrease in body weight, mainly decreased body fat	100
Postprandial fullness	common
Malabsorption	common
Fat (steatorrhoea)	
Iron (anaemia)	
Ca	
Ascorbic acid	
Vit D (osteomalacia)	
Dumping	
Early (faintness and abdominal pain within 10–20 mins of eating)	20–30
Late (hypoglycaemia 2–3 h after eating)	
Diarrhoea (secondary to bile salts; altered motility, bacterial overgrowth)	20
Vomiting (biliary reflux, jejunal distention)	5–15
Oesophageal stricture, secondary biliary reflux	10–15

Unanswered Questions

Further studies and longer term follow-up are needed in order to address questions such as whether prophylactic gastrectomy extends life expectancy and whether there is an increased incidence of cancers at other sites. Another important research question is whether or not surveillance can be improved so that prophylactic surgery can be obviated. This might include a role for optical endoscopic techniques such as coherence tomography, which enables biopsies to be targeted to the area at risk. Alternatively, the development of molecular markers for gastric brushings or for lavage fluid might be an alternative way to overcome the sampling bias inherent in the current random biopsy sampling methods.

Should Identification and Care of These Cases Be in a Specialist Centre?

In order to make any impact upon the morbidity and mortality from HDGC, identification of the families that could potentially benefit from prophylactic gastrectomy will require a careful determination of family history in addition to CDH1 mutation analysis of at-risk individuals. This process requires careful counselling, as already discussed, and the genetic testing needs to be accurate and reproducible with confirmation by a clinical laboratory. Furthermore, the low yield from surveillance, and the high surgical risk of gastrectomy, suggests that these procedures should be performed in specialist centres with expertise in these areas. Since the counselling and clinical care should be separate from the research laboratory, the testing centre should ideally have the research and clinical expertise in one specialist centre to provide the most up-to-date information. For genetic counselling purposes, the patients and families should be provided with information on current research developments in a timely manner while learning more about the management recommendations as they are refined in the future. The genetic counselling or health professional group will thus provide the active link between the research and clinical groups caring for each family.

In view of the need for longitudinal follow-up data and for ongoing research into this condition, families undergoing germline E-cadherin testing should be entered into research protocols for the initial mutational analysis. Patients should also be asked whether they are willing to be entered into a co-operative registry for ongoing research and discovery. A multidisciplinary study focused on HDGC and E-cadherin would ultimately benefit both the families with identified E-cadherin mutations and the research community as a whole. For such studies it is anticipated that each participating research laboratory will develop specific informed consent documents in accordance with the requirements of their institution.

The establishment of specialist centres with the necessary research and clinical expertise should enable considerable progress to be made in this important area. Such research efforts will have long-term implications for improving our understanding and management of sporadic as well as familial gastric cancers.

Acknowledgements

The authors would like to thank Christine Fox for her help with the manuscript preparation. Rebecca Fitzgerald is funded by the MRC and Carlos Caldas by Cancer Research UK.

References

1 Boyle P: Global cancer burden. Lancet 1997; 349:23–26.
2 Msika S, Tazi MA, Benhamiche AM, Couillault C, Harb M, Faivre J: Population-based study of diagnosis, treatment and prognosis of gastric cancer. Br J Surg 1997;84:1474–1478.
3 Allgayer H, Keiss MM, Schildberg FW: Prognostic factors in gastric cancer. Br J Surg 1997; 84:1651–1664.
4 Hisamichi S, Fukai A, Tsubono Y: Evaluation of mass screening for stomach cancer; in Nishi M, et al (eds): Gastric Cancer. Tokyo, Springer-Verlag, 1993 pp 16–25.
5 Parsonnet FG, Vandersteen DP, et al: Helicobacter pylori infection and the risk of gastric carcinoma. N Engl J Med 1991;325:1127–1271.
6 Danesh J: Is Helicobacter pylori infection a cause of gastric neoplasia. Cancer Surveys 1999;33:263–289.
7 Group IAfRCW: Monographs on the evaluation of the carcinogenic risks to humans: Scistosomes Liver Flukes and Helicobacter pylori. 1994, pp 177–241.
8 Vasen HF, Wijnen JT, Menko FH, Kleibeuker JH, Taal BG, Griffioen G, Nagengast FM, Meijers-Heijboer EH, Bertario L, Varesco L, Bisgaard ML, Mohr J, Fodde R, Khan PM: Cancer risk in families with hereditary nonpolyposis colorectal cancer diagnosed by mutation analysis. Gastroenterology 1996;110: 1020–1027.
9 Keller G, Rudelius M, Vogelsang H, Grimm V, Wilhelm MG, Mueller J, Siewert JR, Hofler H: Microsatellite instability and loss of heterozygosity in gastric carcinoma in comparison to family history. Am J Pathol 1998;152:1281–1289.
10 Varley JM, McGown G, Thorncroft M, Tricker KJ, Teare MD, Santibanez-Koref MF, Martin J, Birch JM, Evans DG: An extended Li-Fraumeni kindred with gastric carcinoma and a codon 175 mutation in TP53. J Med Genet 1995;32:942–945.
11 La Vecchia C, Negri E, Franceschi S, Gentile A: Family history and the risk of stomach and colorectal cancer. Cancer 1992;70:50–55.
12 Sokoloff B: Predisposition to cancer in the Bonaparte family. Am J Surg 1938;40:673–678.
13 Guilford P, Hopkins J, Harraway J, McLeod M, McLeod N, Harawira P, Taite H, Scoular R, Miller A, Reeve AE: E-cadherin germline mutations in familial gastric cancer. Nature 1998; 392:402–405.
14 Becker KF, Atkinson MJ, Reich U, Becker I, Nekarda H, Siewert JR, Hofler H: E-cadherin gene mutations provide clues to diffuse type gastric carcinomas. Cancer Res 1994;54:3845–3852.
15 Becker KF, Hofler H: Frequent somatic allelic inactivation of the E-cadherin gene in gastric carcinomas. J Natl Cancer Inst 1995;87:1082–1084.
16 Machado JC, Soares P, Carneiro F, Rocha A, Beck S, Blin N, Berx G: Sobrinho-Simoes M: E-cadherin gene mutations provide a genetic basis for the phenotypic divergence of mixed gastric carcinomas. Lab Invest 1999;79:459–465.
17 Oda T, Kanai Y, Oyama T, Yoshiura K, Shimoyama Y, Birchmeier W, Sugimura T, Hirohashi S: E-cadherin gene mutations in human gastric carcinoma cell lines. Proc Natl Acad Sci USA 1994;91:1858–1862.
18 Perl AK, Wilgenbus P, Dahl U, Semb H, Christofori G: A causal role for E-cadherin in the transition from adenoma to carcinoma. Nature 1998;392:190–193.
19 Yoshiura K, Kanai Y, Ochiai A, Shimoyama Y, Sugimura T, Hirohashi S: Silencing of the E-cadherin invasion-suppressor gene by CpG methylation in human carcinomas. Proc Natl Acad Sci U S A 1995;92:7416–7419.
20 Guilford PJ, Hopkins JB, Grady WM, Markowitz SD, Willis J, Lynch H, Rajput A, Wiesner GL, Lindor NM, Burgart LJ, Toro TT, Lee D, Limacher JM, Shaw DW, Findlay MP, Reeve AE: E-cadherin germline mutations define an inherited cancer syndrome dominated by diffuse gastric cancer. Hum Mutat 1999;14:249–255.

21 Caldas C, Carneiro F, Lynch HT, Yokota J, Wiesner GL, Powell SM, Lewis FR, Huntsman DG, Pharoah PD, Jankowski JA, MacLeod P, Vogelsang H, Keller G, Park KG, Richards FM, Maher ER, Gayther SA, Oliveira C, Grehan N, Wight D, Seruca R, Roviello F, Ponder BA, Jackson CE: Familial gastric cancer: overview and guidelines for management. J Med Genet 1999;36:873–880.
22 IGCLC: First Worskshop of the International Gastric Cancer Linkage Consortium (IGCLC). Cambridge, University of Cambridge, 1999.
23 Iida S, Akiyama Y, Ichikawa W, Yamashita T, Nomizu T, Nihei Z, Sugihara K, Yuasa Y: Infrequent germ-line mutation of the E-cadherin gene in Japanese familial gastric cancer kindreds. Clin Cancer Res 1999;5:1445–1447.
24 Avizienyte E, Launonen V, Salovaara R, Kiviluoto T, Aaltonen LA: E-cadherin is not frequently mutated in hereditary gastric cancer. J Med Genet 2001;38:49–52.
25 Yoon KA, Ku JL, Yang HK, Kim WH, Park SY, Park JG: Germline mutations of E-cadherin gene in Korean familial gastric cancer patients. J Hum Genet 1999;44:177–180.
26 Gayther SA, Gorringe KL, Ramus SJ, Huntsman D, Roviello F, Grehan N, Machado JC, Pinto E, Seruca R, Halling K, MacLeod P, Powell SM, Jackson CE, Ponder BA, Caldas C: Identification of germ-line E-cadherin mutations in gastric cancer families of European origin. Cancer Res 1998;58:4086–4089.
27 Pharoah PD, Guilford P, Caldas C: Incidence of gastric cancer and breast cancer in CDH1 (E-cadherin) mutation carriers from hereditary diffuse gastric cancer families. Gastroenterology 2001;121:1348–1353.
28 Richards FM, McKee SA, Rajpar MH, Cole TR, Evans DG, Jankowski JA, McKeown C, Sanders DS, Maher ER: Germline E-cadherin gene (CDH1) mutations predispose to familial gastric cancer and colorectal cancer. Hum Mol Genet 1999;8:607–610.
29 Oliveira C, Bordin MC, Grehan N, Huntsman DG, Gianpaolo S, Machado JC, Kiviluoto TA, Aaltonen L, Jackson CE, Seruca R, Caldas C: Screening E-Cadherin in gastric cancer families reveals germ-line mutations only in hereditary diffuse gastric cancer kindred. Hum Mut 2001, in press.
30 Berx G, Becker KF, Hofler H, van Roy F: Mutations of the human E-cadherin (CDH1) gene. Hum Mutat 1998;12:226–237.
31 Grady WM, Willis J, Guilford PJ, Dunbier AK, Toro TT, Lynch H, Wiesner G, Ferguson K, Eng C, Park JG, Kim SJ, Markowitz S: Methylation of the CDH1 promoter as the second genetic hit in hereditary diffuse gastric cancer. Nat Genet 2000;26:16–17.
32 Graff JR, Herman JG, Lapidus RG, Chopra H, Xu R, Jarrard DF, Isaacs WB, Pitha PM, Davidson NE, Baylin SB: E-cadherin expression is silenced by DNA hypermethylation in human breast and prostate carcinomas. Cancer Res 1995;55:5195–5199.
33 Graff JR, Greenberg VE, Herman JG, Westra WH, Boghaert ER, Ain KB, Saji M, Zeiger MA, Zimmer SG, Baylin SB: Distinct patterns of E-cadherin CpG island methylation in papillary, follicular, Hurthle's cell, poorly differentiated human thyroid carcinoma. Cancer Res 1998; 58:2063–2066.
34 Machado JC, Oliveira C, Carvalho R, Soares P, Berx G, Caldas C, Seruca R, Carneiro F, Sobrinho-Simoes M: E-cadherin gene (CDH1) promoter methylation as the second hit in sporadic diffuse gastric carcinoma. Oncogene 2001;20:1525–1528.
35 Fang J, Xiao S: Alteration of DNA methylation in gastrointestinal carcinogenesis. J Gastroenterol Hepatol 2001;16:960–968.
36 Kintner C: Regulation of embryonic cell adhesion by the cadherin cytoplasmic domain. Cell 1992;69:225–236.
37 Bracke ME, Roy FM, Mareel MM: The E-cadherin/catenin complex in invasion and metastasis. Curr Top Microbiol Imm 1996;213:123–161.
38 Nigam AK, Savage FJ, Boulos PB, Stamp GW, Liu D, Pignatelli M: Loss of cell-cell and cell-matrix adhesion molecules in colorectal cancer. Br J Cancer 1993;68:507–514.
39 Kinsella AR, Lepts GC, Hill CL, Jones M: Reduced E-cadherin expression correlates with increased invasiveness in colorectal carcinoma cell lines. Clin Exp Metastasis 1994;12:335–342.
40 Berx G, Cleton-Jansen AM, Nollet F, de Leeuw WJ, van de Vijver M, Cornelisse C, van Roy F: E-cadherin is a tumour/invasion suppressor gene mutated in human lobular breast cancers. EMBO J 1995;14:6107–6115.
41 Frixen UH, Behrens J, Sachs M, Eberle G, Voss B, Warda A, Lochner D, Birchmeier W: E-cadherin-mediated cell-cell adhesion prevents invasiveness of human carcinoma cells. J Cell Biol 1991;113:173–185.
42 Jones EG: Familial gastric cancer. NZ Med J 1964;63:287–296.
43 Keller G, Vogelsang H, Becker I, Hutter J, Ott K, Candidus S, Grundei T, Becker KF, Mueller J, Siewert JR, Hofler H: Diffuse type gastric and lobular breast carcinoma in a familial gastric cancer patient with an E-cadherin germline mutation. Am J Pathol 1999;155:337–342.
44 Eurogast SG: An international association between Helicobacter pylori infection and gastric cancer. Lancet 1993;341:1359–1362.
45 Kikuchi S, Wada O, Nakajima T, Nishi T, Kobayashi O, Konishi T, Inaba Y: Serum anti-Helicobacter pylori antibody and gastric carcinoma among young adults. Research Group on Prevention of Gastric Carcinoma among Young Adults. Cancer 1995;75:2789–2793.
46 Campbell S, Fraser A, Holliss B, Schmid J, O'Toole PW: Evidence for ethnic tropism of Helicobacter pylori. Infect Immun 1997;65: 3708–3712.
47 Salahshor S, Hou H, Diep CB, Loukola A, Zhang H, Liu T, Chen J, Iselius L, Rubio C, Lothe RA, Aaltonen L, Sun XF, Lindmark G, Lindblom A: A germline E-cadherin mutation in a family with gastric and colon cancer. Int J Mol Med 2001;8:439–443.
48 Huntsman DG, Carneiro F, Lewis FR, MacLeod PM, Hayashi A, Monaghan KG, Maung R, Seruca R, Jackson CE, Caldas C: Early gastric cancer in young, asymptomatic carriers of germ-line E-cadherin mutations. N Engl J Med 2001;344:1904–1909.
49 Chun YS, Lindor NM, Smyrk TC, Petersen BT, Burgart LJ, Guilford PJ, Donohue JH: Germline: E-cadherin gene mutations: is prophylactic total gastrectomy indicated? Cancer 2001;92:181–187.
50 Lewis FR, Mellinger JD, Hayashi A, Lorelli D, Monaghan KG, Carneiro F, Huntsman DG, Jackson CE, Caldas C: Prophylactic total gastrectomy for familial gastric cancer. Surgery 2001;130:612–617; discussion 617–619.
51 Khurana K, Loosman A, Numann P, Khan S: Prophylactic mastectomy: pathologic findings in high-risk patients. Arch Pathol Lab Med 2000;124:378–381.
52 Lu KH, Garber JE, Cramer DW, Welch WR, Niloff J, Schrag D, Berkowitz RS, Muto MG: Occult ovarian tumors in women with BRCA1 or BRCA2 mutations undergoing prophylactic oophorectomy. J Clin Oncol 2000;18:2728–2732.
53 Miholic J, Meyer HJ, Kotzerke J, Balks J, Aebert H, Jahne J, Weimann A, Pichlmayr R: Emptying of the gastric substitute after total gastrectomy. Jejunal interposition versus Roux-y esophagojejunostomy. Ann Surg 1989; 210:165–172.
54 Miholic J, Meyer HJ, Muller MJ, Weimann A, Pichlmayr R: Nutritional consequences of total gastrectomy: the relationship between mode of reconstruction, postprandial symptoms, body composition. Surgery 1990;108:488–494.
55 Cuschieri A: Jejunal pouch reconstruction after total gastrectomy for cancer: experience in 29 patients. Br J Surg 1990;77:421–424.

Review Article

Digestive Diseases

Dig Dis 2002;20:32–37

Chronic Pancreatitis and Pancreatic Cancer

Patrick Maisonneuve[a] Albert B. Lowenfels[b]

[a]Division of Epidemiology and Biostatistics, European Institute of Oncology, Milan, Italy and [b]Departments of Surgery and Community and Preventive Medicine, New York, Medical College, Valhalla, N.Y., USA

Key Words
Pancreatitis · Pancreatic cancer · Risk factors · Prevention · Tobacco smoking

Abstract
Pancreatic cancer is the fourth leading cause of cancer deaths in the USA in both sexes. Early diagnosis is difficult and the overall mortality rate is high. Individuals at high risk for pancreatic cancer include smokers, and persons with all forms of chronic alcoholic, metabolic, tropical or hereditary pancreatitis. The duration of exposure to inflammation seems to be the major factor involved in the transition from benign to malignant condition. Smoking, which appears to further accelerate the carcinogenic transformation, remains the strongest risk factor amenable to preventive intervention.

Introduction

Pancreatic cancer is the fourth leading cause of cancer death in the USA in both sexes [1] and among the top cancer killers in most developed countries [2]. The very low survival reflects the fact that this neoplasm is usually diagnosed in an incurable stage and highlights the need for early detection or prevention. Still, knowledge of risk factors and understanding of carcinogenic mechanisms are crucial elements in the setting of any intervention strategy.

Smoking is the most established risk factor for pancreatic cancer and is responsible for one third of all tumors. Smokers have a two- to three-fold increased risk compared to non-smokers and the risk remains elevated for one or two decades after cessation of smoking. There is no epidemiological evidence that alcohol consumption is associated with pancreatic cancer. High caloric intake, high fat diet and high consumption of cured meat has been associated with an increased risk of pancreas cancer, but overall, diet is responsible for no more than 20% of all tumors. Finally benign conditions such as pancreatitis or diabetes are responsible for a very small fraction of tumors (<5%) and about 10% of cancers are of familial origin [3]. Still, the etiology of a large proportion of pancreatic cancers is unknown and better knowledge of the steps and factors involved in the transition from benign to malignant disease would be of major help for both its prevention and treatment. This article will focus on the association between pancreatitis and pancreatic cancer.

Supported by Grants from the Italian Association for Cancer Research, the C. D. Smithers Foundation, Inc, and Solvay Pharmaceuticals.

KARGER
Fax + 41 61 306 12 34
E-Mail karger@karger.ch
www.karger.com

0257–2753/02/0201–0032$18.50/0

Accessible online at:
www.karger.com/journals/ddi

Dr. P. Maisonneuve
PM Division of Epidemiology and Biostatistics, European Institute of Oncology
Via Ripamonti 435
I–20141 Milan (Italy)
Fax +39 02 57489822, Fax +39 02 57489813, E-Mail patrick.maisonneuve@ieo.it

Inflammation and Cancer

The association between chronic inflammation and certain malignancies has been recognized for many years. Already in 1863, the German pathologist Rudolf Virchow noted leucocytes in neoplastic tissues and made a connection between inflammation and cancer. Most of the early data were derived from descriptions of chronic cutaneous lesions, such as ulcers, burn scars or draining sinus tract [4, 5]. Since then, the association between chronic inflammation and subsequent cancer has been recognized in many conditions (bladder cancer after schistosomiasis, ovarian cancer after pelvic inflammatory disease, esophageal cancer after Barrett's metaplasia, colorectal cancer after inflammatory bowel disease, ulcerative colitis and Crohn's disease, lung cancer and mesothelioma after silicosis or asbestosis and finally pancreas cancer after chronic pancreatitis). Inflammatory process is also an important cofactor in viral carcinogenesis (gastric cancer and MALT lymphoma after *H. pylori*, cervical cancer after papillomavirus, liver cancer after hepatitis B and C virus and Kaposi sarcoma after human herpes virus type 8 infection) [6].

Acute Pancreatitis

Acute pancreatitis may result from a wide variety of causes with gallstones and alcohol responsible for 60–80% of all cases [7]. It occurs suddenly, lasts generally for a short period of time and usually resolves. Some people have more than one attack and recover completely after each, but acute pancreatitis can be a severe, life-threatening illness with many complications. Nevertheless, single attacks of acute pancreatitis are not believed to be associated with increased risk of pancreatic cancer, unless evolving into recurrent chronic pancreatitis.

Chronic Pancreatitis

Chronic pancreatitis is a complex disease, resulting of fibroinflammatory changes in the pancreas from various causes. It is an irreversible process with permanent loss of pancreatic function. Alcohol is the major cause of chronic pancreatitis, with disease going through phases of recurrent acute pancreatitis. Other etiologies include tropical pancreatitis, metabolic pancreatitis, hereditary pancreatitis, vasculitis, congenital defects such as cystic fibrosis, some infectious diseases, drugs and radiation therapy. Yet, chronic pancreatitis remains idiopathic in a significant group of patients [8].

The association between chronic pancreatitis and ductal adenocarcinoma of the pancreas was discussed already in 1913 by John B. Deaver who wrote: 'It may not be out of place here to record my belief that carcinoma of the pancreas is in many instances brought into existence by previous pancreatitis. This is in line with the known fact that chronic irritation predispose to cancer as is seen in 'chimney-sweep' cancer, 'pipe' cancer of the lip, ulcus carcinomatosum of the stomach, cancer of the gall-bladder with gall-stones and many other forms of the disease elsewhere' [9].

There have been many early case reports linking the two diseases, but it is difficult to tell whether these two instances might have arisen by chance, or whether the pancreatitis is caused by ductal obstruction from the cancer. In fact, pancreatic cancer is occasionally found at operation in patients originally diagnosed with chronic pancreatitis and pancreatitis is present at diagnosis of pancreatic cancer in a small proportion of patients [10–12].

Early studies on pancreas cancer did not identify pancreatitis as a significant risk factor [13–17]. In 1973, in a hospital-based case-control study, Wynder et al. [18] found an excess of pancreatitis (4 cases and no controls) but further investigations show that 3 of the pancreatic conditions were found concurrently with the cancer. In 1990, Farrow et al. [19] found 5 cases and no controls with a history of pancreatitis at least 3 years before the diagnosis of pancreatic cancer. Similar results were found in a series of successive case-control studies [20–24]. In 1993, Lowenfels et al. [25] undertook a multi-center historical cohort study of 2015 subjects with chronic pancreatitis, recruited from clinical centers in six countries. For subjects with a minimum of two years of follow-up the risk of pancreatic cancer was 16.5-fold higher than that of the general population. The risk appeared to be independent of sex, country, and type of pancreatitis. These results were confirmed by Talamini et al. [26] who still found significant increased risk considering only cancer arising 5 or more years after the diagnosis of CP.

Hereditary Pancreatitis

Hereditary pancreatitis (HP) is a rare pancreatic disorder, accounting for approximately 1% of all reported cases of pancreatitis. It was first identified by Comfort and Steinberg in 1952 [27]. The symptoms, signs and disease course resemble that of other forms of pancreatitis but the onset of the disease occurs at an early age, often in childhood, with multiple members of the family afflicted. It is inherited in autosomal dominant fashion, with an estimated 80% phenotypic penetrance, and is seen in various ethnic groups. Two different mutations in the cationic trypsinogen gene (R122H, N29I) have been identified so far in 60–70% of kindreds [28–33].

Two large independent epidemiological studies, the International Hereditary Pancreatitis Study Group and the European Registry of Hereditary Pancreatitis and Pancreatic Cancer (EUROPAC), have calculated an approximately 50- to 70-fold increased risk of pancreatic cancer in patients with HP [34–35]. In both studies, the risk of cancer started to rise between age 40 and 50, and the cumulative incidence of cancer reached 40% after 70 years of age. In the report by Lowenfels et al. [34] the cumulative incidence reached 70% in patients with paternal inheritance, suggesting genetic imprinting. Other groups have subsequently reported pancreatic tumors in HP patients with both paternal and maternal inheritance [35–37]. Pancreatic cancer has been reported in kindreds with R122H mutations, N29I mutations or no identifiable gene mutations in the setting of an obvious HP phenotype [34–35].

Tropical Pancreatitis

Tropical pancreatitis (TCP) and fibrocalculous pancreatic diabetes (FCPD) are rare forms of chronic pancreatitis occurring in tropical and subtropical regions and characterized by pancreatic calculi, diabetes and abdominal pain. In FCPD diabetes is the first major clinical sign leading to diagnosis. These diseases are most prevalent in southern India and sub-Sahara Africa [38]. It generally affects children between 12 and 15 years old. Family history is uncommon The etiology of TCP and FCDP remains unknown despite efforts to identify environmental factors or genetic factors such as the PRSS1/ R122H mutation, as seen in hereditary pancreatitis [39–40].

As in hereditary pancreatitis, pancreas cancer is a common complication in tropical pancreatitis. Augustine and Ramesh reported high incidence of cancer (8.3%) in patients with TCP, in contrast with the low incidence of pancreatic cancer in southern India [41]. In the study by Chari et al. [42], 6 of 185 patients with TCP followed for an average of 4.5 years died from cancer of the pancreas (RR = 100; 95% CI = 37–218). The risk was still high when restricted to the 3 biospy-proven cancer and applying more stringent assumptions on the background cancer rates (RR = 5.0, 95% CI = 1.0–14.6). Few subsequent reports confirmed the high risk of pancreas cancer in TCP and FCPD [43–44].

Cystic Fibrosis

Cystic fibrosis (CF) constitutes the most common life-threatening autosomal-recessive disorder in the white population affecting approximately 25,000 children and adults in the United States. CF causes the body to produce an abnormally thick, sticky mucus, due to the faulty transport of sodium and chloride (salt) within cells lining organs such as the lungs and pancreas, to their outer surfaces. The thick CF mucus also obstructs the pancreas, preventing enzymes from reaching the intestines to help break down and digest food. More than 1000 different mutations in the Cystic Fibrosis Trans-membrane Conductance Regulator gene (CFTR) have been identified so far. The most common is ΔF_{508}, which is present in 70–80% of patients with CF.

The phenotypic spectrum associated with different mutations is very large, comprising obstructive azoospermia, disseminated bronchiectasis and chronic sinusitis. The majority of CF patients suffer from pancreatic insufficiency which usually begins in early childhood but episodes of pancreatitis are common in subjects with preserved exocrine pancreatic function [45]. In fact, many idiopathic pancreatitis patients have compound heterozygote genotypes in which both copies of the CFTR gene are abnormal. In these patients, the pancreatic disease can be viewed as a mild variant of cystic fibrosis, in which there is sufficient residual CFTR function to prevent lung disease [46]. With improved survival and identification of new mutations responsible for less severe forms of cystic fibrosis, the proportion of adult patients with CF has increased substantially in the last years, and concern about cancer risk is rising [47].

Several case reports described patients with CF and adenocarcinomas of the pancreas [48–52]. In 1995, Neglia et al. [53] performed a retrospective cohort study of the occurrence of cancer in 28,511 CF patients from 1985 through 1992 in the USA and Canada. They also analyzed proportional incidence ratios to assess the association between specific cancers and CF in Europe and found consistently on both continents increased risk of digestive tract tumors, but the absolute risk is very small.

Risk Factors for Pancreas Cancer in Patients with Pancreatitis

Several case-control studies have established that the risk of chronic pancreatitis was associated with both alcohol intake and cigarette consumption, and that their effects are independent [54, 55]. In particular, Lin et al. [55] found that cigarette smoking was associated with a 7.8-fold risk of developing chronic pancreatitis after adjustment for ethanol intake and other major risk factors. Cavallini et al. [56] demonstrated that smoking was associated with the development of calcifications. The mean time to onset of calcification was 8 years in smokers against 12 years in nonsmokers. Imoto et al. [57] found similar results in a subset of patients with late-onset idiopathic chronic pancreatitis. In an animal model, Hartwig et al. [58] demonstrated that ethanol induces pancreatic ischemia and that cigarette smoke potentiates the amount of pancreatic injury generated by ethanol alone.

As smoking is also a major risk factor for pancreatic cancer, it could appear as a potential confounder in the association between pancreatitis and pancreatic cancer. In particular, in cohort studies, the rate of pancreatic cancer in patients with pancreatitis is compared to the rate of pancreatic cancer in the background population. Since patients with pancreatitis are more likely to be heavy drinkers and smokers, then the excess of pancreatic cancer could just be due to smoking [59]. Still the association between pancreatic cancer and pancreatitis has been confirmed in other study designs, unbiased in regard of smoking.

Of interest, Lowenfels et al. [60] in a recent report, provided information on smoking as an additional risk factor in hereditary pancreatitis. As in the general population, smoking doubles the risk of pancreatic cancer and accounts for approximately 25–30% of all pancreatic tumors. In addition, in his cohort pancreatic cancer developed in average 20 years earlier in smokers than in nonsmokers.

Early Diagnosis

Chronic pancreatitis causes destruction of the pancreatic gland, leading to tissue fibrosis and hyperplasia. Brat et al. [61] described three cases in which atypical papillary hyperplasia of the pancreas preceded for a period of 17 months to 10 years the development of an infiltrating adenocarcinoma of the pancreas, supporting the concept that there is a stepwise progression from intraductal hyperplasia to infiltrating carcinoma of the pancreas. These lesions, called Pancreatic Intraepithelial Neoplasia (PanIN), harbour a number of well-characterised genetic alterations. In contrast to precursor lesions in carcinoma of the uterine cervix, colon or breast, these preneoplastic lesions of the pancreas are not clinically easily recognizable. Likewise, there is no reliable molecular or genetic testing available so far for the detection of pancreatic dysplasia.

Mutations in the k-ras oncogene are rare events in normal pancreas [62] but are present in the majority (80%) of pancreatic cancer [63]. k-ras mutations have also been detected in a small proportion of patients with chronic pancreatitis [64]. Lüttges et al. [65] show that ductal lesions in patients with CP exhibit k-ras mutations without additional indications of neoplastic transformation such as severe dysplasia or mutated p53 protein. Therefore in our current knowledge, the detection of k-ras mutations in CP patients could not alone predict neoplastic transformation, but long term follow-up of these patients would provide important clues.

Prevention and Screening

In its guide to clinical preventive services, the U.S. Preventive Services Task Force stated that: 'Routine screening for pancreatic cancer in asymptomatic persons, using abdominal palpation, ultrasonography, or serologic markers, is not recommended. All patients should be counseled regarding use of tobacco products. Counseling to reduce fat and cholesterol intake and to increase intake of fruits and vegetables may be recommended on other grounds' [66]. Still screening for pancreatic cancer in high risk individuals is questionable. During the Third International Symposium on Inherited Diseases of the Pancreas, consensus guidelines for prevention, screening and treatment of pancreatic cancer in patients with hereditary pancreatitis were drawn by an international experts committee [67]. The guidelines indicate that, whilst no screening protocol has proven to be effective in any cohort at risk of pancreatic cancer, minimally invasive imaging screening could be offered in patients with the HP phenotype beginning at the age of 40 years. Optimally, screening should be performed within multi-center Institutional Review Board-approved protocols. Members of HP kindreds should be counseled at a young age to avoid smoking and current smokers should be encourage to stop smoking. Finally every attempt should be made to identify and eliminate concomitant risk factors for recurrent acute and chronic pancreatitis such as alcohol intake.

Conclusion

Consistent epidemiologic evidence confirms the association between antecedent chronic pancreatitis and pancreatic cancer. Additional evidence comes from pathologic studies where a gradual progression from normal tissue to hyperplasia and eventually pancreatic cancer has been observed. Cancer risk is higher in patients where pancreatitis begins early in life, such as in hereditary or tropical pancreatitis suggesting that the duration of exposure to chronic inflammation is a major factor. Smoking, which is associated with pancreatitis risk and severity as well as pancreatic cancer risk further advances the age at which cancer develops. Smoking remains the strongest risk factor amenable to preventive intervention and should be proscribed in patients with pancreatitis and in members of hereditary pancreatitis families.

References

1 Greenlee RT, Hill-Harmon MB, Murray T, Thun M: Cancer statistics, 2001. CA Cancer J Clin 2001;51:15–36.
2 Pisani P, Parkin DM, Bray F, Ferlay J: Estimates of the worldwide mortality from 25 cancers in 1990. Int J Cancer 1999;83:18–29.
3 Simon B, Printz H: Epidemiological trends in pancreatic neoplasias. Dig Dis 2001;19:6–14.
4 Treves N, Pack GT: The development of cancer in burn scars. Surg Gynecol Obstet 1930;51:749.
5 Bereston ES, Ney C: Squamous cell carcinoma arising in a chronic osteomyelitic sinus tract with metastasis. Arch Surg 1941;43:257.
6 Balkwill F, Mantovani A: Inflammation and cancer: back to Virchow? Lancet 2001;357:539–545.
7 Steinberg W, Tenner S: Acute pancreatitis. N Engl J Med 1994;330:1198–1210.
8 Steer ML, Waxman I, Freedman S: Chronic pancreatitis. N Engl J Med.;332:1482–1490.
9 Deaver JB: Pancreatic lymphangitis and chronic pancreatitis. JAMA 1913;60:1–4.
10 Vickers SM, Chan C, Heslin MJ, Bartolucci A, Aldrete JS: The role of pancreaticoduodenectomy in the treatment of severe chronic pancreatitis. Am Surg 1999;65:1108–1112.
11 Deixonne B, Pignodel C, Chazelet C, Joujoux JM, Raffanel C, Baumel H: Small carcinomas of the pancreas with associated chronic pancreatitis: two case reports. Eur J Surg Oncol 1989;15:265–270.
12 Wharton SM, Rahman Z, Johnson CD: Missed curable carcinoma of the pancreas presenting as chronic pancreatitis. Postgrad Med J 1997;73:577–579.
13 Appel MF: Hereditary pancreatitis. Review and presentation of an additional kindred. Arch Surg 1974;108:63–65.
14 Haines A, Moss A, Whittemore AS, Quivey J: A case-control study of pancreatic carcinoma. J Cancer Res Clin Oncol 1982;103:93–97.
15 Gold EB, Gordis L, Diener MD, Seltser R, Boitnott JK, Bynum TE, Hutcheon DF: Diet and other risk factors for cancer of the pancreas. Cancer 1985;55:460–467.
16 Mack TM, Peters JM, Yu MC, Hanisch R, Wright WE, Henderson BE: Pancreas cancer is unrelated to the workplace in Los Angeles. Am J Ind Med 1985;7:253–266.
17 Bueno de Mesquita HB, Maisonneuve P, Moerman CJ, Walker AM: Aspects of medical history and exocrine carcinoma of the pancreas: A population-based case-control study in the Netherlands. Int J Cancer 1992;52:17–23.
18 Wynder EL, Mabuchi K, Maruchi N, Fortner J: A case-control study of cancer of the pancreas. Cancer 1973;31:641–648.
19 Farrow DC, Davis S: Risk of pancreatic cancer in relation to medical history and use of tobacco, alcohol and coffee. Int J Cancer 1990;45:816–820.
20 Howe GR, Jain M, Miller AB: Dietary factors and risk of pancreatic cancer: Results of a Canadian population-based case-control study. Int J Cancer 1990;45:604–608.
21 Kalapothaki V, Tzonou A, Hsieh CC, Toupadaki N, Karakatsani A, Trichopoulos D: Tobacco, ethanol, coffee, pancreatitis, diabetes mellitus, and cholelithiasis as risk factors for pancreatic carcinoma. Cancer Causes Control 1993;4:375–382.
22 Fernandez E, La Vecchia C, Porta M, Negri E, D'Avanzo B, Boyle P: Pancreatitis and the risk of pancreatic cancer. Pancreas 1995;11:185–189.
23 Bansal P, Sonnenberg A: Pancreatitis is a risk factor for pancreatic cancer. Gastroenterology 1995;109:247–251.
24 Ekbom A, McLaughlin JK, Karlsson BM, Nyren O, Gridley G, Adami HO, Fraumeni JF: Pancreatitis and pancreatic cancer: a population-based study. J Natl Cancer Inst 1994;86:625–627.
25 Lowenfels AB, Maisonneuve P, Cavallini G, Ammann RW, Lankisch PG, Andersen JR, Dimagno EP, Andren SA, Domellof L: Pancreatitis and the risk of pancreatic cancer. International Pancreatitis Study Group. N Engl J Med 1993;328:1433–1437.
26 Talamini G, Falconi M, Bassi C, Sartori N, Salvia R, Caldiron E, Frulloni L, Di Francesco V, Vaona B, Bovo P, Vantini I, Pederzoli P, Cavallini G: Incidence of cancer in the course of chronic pancreatitis. Am J Gastroenterol 1999;94:1253–1260.
27 Comfort M, Steinberg A: Pedigree of a family with hereditary chronic relapsing pancreatitis. Gastroenterology 1952;21:54–63.
28 Whitcomb DC, Gorry MC, Preston RA, Furey W, Sossenheimer MJ, Ulrich CD, Martin SP, Gates LK Jr, Amann ST, Toskes PP, Liddle R, McGrath K, Uomo G, Post JC, Ehrlich GD: Hereditary pancreatitis is caused by a mutation in the cationic trypsinogen gene. Nat Genet 1996;14:141–145.
29 Howes N, Greenhalf W, Rutherford S, O'Donnell M, Mountford R, Ellis I, Whitcomb D, Imrie C, Drumm B, Neoptolemos JP: A new polymorphism for the RI22H mutation in hereditary pancreatitis. Gut 2001;48:247–250.
30 Gorry MC, Gabbaizedeh D, Furey W, Gates LK, Preston RA, Aston CE, Zhang Y, Ulrich CD, Ehrlich GD, Whitcomb DC: Mutations in the cationic trypsinogen gene are associated with recurrent acute and chronic pancreatitis. Gastroenterology 1997;113:1063–1068.
31 Applebaum-Shapiro SE, Finch R, Pfützer RH, Hepp LA, Gates L, Amann S, Martin S, Ulrich CD, Whitcomb DC: Hereditary pancreatitis in North America: The Pittsburgh-Midwest Multi-Center Pancreatic Study Group study. Pancreatology 2001;1:439–443.
32 Nishimori I, Kamakura M, Fujikawa-Adachi K, Morita M, Onishi S, Yokoyama K, Makino I, Ishida H, Yamamoto M, Watanabe S, Ogawa M: Mutations in exons 2 and 3 of the cationic trypsinogen gene in Japanese families with hereditary pancreatitis. Gut 1999;44:259–263.
33 Sahin-Toth M, Toth M: Gain-of-function mutations associated with hereditary pancreatitis enhance autoactivation of human cationic trypsinogen. Biochem Biophys Res Commun 2000;278:286–289.
34 Lowenfels AB, Maisonneuve P, DiMagno EP, Elitsur Y, Gates LK Jr, Perrault J, Whitcomb DC: Hereditary pancreatitis and the risk of pancreatic cancer. International Hereditary Pancreatitis Study Group. J Natl Cancer Inst 1997;89:442–446.
35 Howes N, Wong T, Greenhalf W, Lerch M, Deviere J, O'Donnell M, Ellis I, Mountford R, Neoptolemos JP for the Consortium of EUROPAC: Pancreatic cancer risk in hereditary pancreatitis in Europe. Digestion 2000;61:300.

36 Lerch MM, Ellis I, Whitcomb DC, Keim V, Simon P, Howes N, Rutherford S, Domschke W, Imrie CW, Neoptolemos JP: Maternal inheritance pattern of hereditary pancreatitis in patients with pancreatic carcinoma. J Natl Cancer Inst 1999;91:723–724.
37 Lowenfels AB, Maisonneuve P: Re: Maternal inheritance pattern of hereditary pancreatitis in patients with pancreatic carcinoma. J Natl Cancer Inst 1999;91:1590–1591.
38 Ramesh H: Tropical pancreatitis.Indian J Gastroenterol 1997;16:20–25.
39 Rossi L, Whitcomb DC, Ehrlich GD, Gorry MC, Parvin S, Sattar S, Ali L, Azad Khan AK, Gyr N: Lack of R117H mutation in the cationic trypsinogen gene in patients with tropical pancreatitis from Bangladesh. Pancreas 1998; 17:278–280.
40 Hassan Z, Mohan V, McDermott MF, Ali L, Ogunkolade WB, Aganna E, Cassell PG, Deepa R, Khan AK, Hitman GA: Pancreatitis in fibrocalculous pancreatic diabetes mellitus is not associated with common mutations in the trypsinogen gene. Diabetes Metab Res Rev 2000;16:454–457.
41 Augustine P, Ramesh H: Is tropical pancreatitis premalignant? Am J Gastroenterol 1992;87: 1005–1008.
42 Chari ST, Mohan V, Pitchumoni CS, Viswanathan M, Madanagopalan N, Lowenfels AB: Risk of pancreatic carcinoma in tropical calcifying pancreatitis: an epidemiologic study. Pancreas 1994;9:62.
43 Das K, Goenka MK, Wig JD, Nagi B, Bhasin D: Pancreatic carcinoma complicating tropical pancreatitis in north India. Indian J Gastroenterol 1996;15:103.
44 Mohan V, Premalatha G, Padma A, Chari ST, Pitchumoni CS: Fibrocalculous pancreatic diabetes. Long-term survival analysis. Diabetes Care 1996;19:1274–1278.
45 Durie PR: Pancreatitis and mutations of the cystic fibrosis gene. N Engl J Med 1998;339: 687–688.
46 Cohn JA, Bornstein JD, Jowell PS: Cystic fibrosis mutations and genetic predisposition to idiopathic chronic pancreatitis. Med Clin North Am 2000;84:621–631.
47 FitzSimmons SC: The changing epidemiology of cystic fibrosis. J Pediatr 1993;122:1–9.
48 Neglia JP, Wielinski CL, Warwick WJ: Cancer risk among patients with cystic fibrosis. J Pediatr 1991;119:764–766.
49 Tedesco FJ, Brown R, Schuman BM: Pancreatic carcinoma in a patient with cystic fibrosis. Gastrointest Endosc 1986;32:25–26.
50 McIntosh JC, Schoumacher RA, Tiller RE: Pancreatic adenocarcinoma in a patient with cystic fibrosis. Am J Med 1988;85:592.
51 Tsongalis GJ, Faber G, Dalldorf FG, Friedman KJ, Silverman LM, Yankaskas JR: Association of pancreatic adenocarcinoma, mild lung disease, and delta F508 mutation in a cystic fibrosis patient.Clin Chem 1994;40:1972–1974.
52 Sheldon CD, Hodson ME, Carpenter LM, Swerdlow AJ: A cohort study of cystic fibrosis and malignancy. Br J Cancer 1993;68:1025–1028.
53 Neglia JP, FitzSimmons SC, Maisonneuve P, Schoni MH, Schoni-Affolter F, Corey M, Lowenfels AB: The risk of cancer among patients with cystic fibrosis. Cystic Fibrosis and Cancer Study Group. N Engl J Med 1995;332:494–499.
54 Talamini G, Bassi C, Falconi M, Sartori N, Salvia R, Rigo L, Castagnini A, Di Francesco V, Frulloni L, Bovo P, Vaona B, Angelini G, Vantini I, Cavallini G, Pederzoli P: Alcohol and smoking as risk factors in chronic pancreatitis and pancreatic cancer. Dig Dis Sci 1999;44: 1303–1311.
55 Lin Y, Tamakoshi A, Hayakawa T, Ogawa M, Ohno Y: Cigarette smoking as a risk factor for chronic pancreatitis: a case-control study in Japan. Research Committee on Intractable Pancreatic Diseases. Pancreas 2000;21:109–114.
56 Cavallini G, Talamini G, Vaona B, Bovo P, Filippini M, Rigo L, Angelini G, Vantini I, Riela A, Frulloni L: Effect of alcohol and smoking on pancreatic lithogenesis in the course of chronic pancreatitis. Pancreas 1994;9:42–46.
57 Imoto M, DiMagno EP: Cigarette smoking increases the risk of pancreatic calcification in late-onset but not early-onset idiopathic chronic pancreatitis. Pancreas 2000;21:115–119.
58 Hartwig W, Werner J, Ryschich E, Mayer H, Schmidt J, Gebhard MM, Herfarth C, Klar E: Cigarette smoke enhances ethanol-induced pancreatic injury. Pancreas 2000;21:272–278.
59 Karlson BM, Ekbom A, Josefsson S, McLaughlin JK, Fraumeni JF, Jr., Nyren O: The risk of pancreatic cancer following pancreatitis: an association due to confounding? Gastroenterology 1997;113:587–592.
60 Lowenfels AB, Maisonneuve P, Whitcomb DC, Lerch MM, DiMagno EP: Cigarette smoking as a risk factor for pancreatic cancer in patients with hereditary pancreatitis. JAMA 2001;286: 169–170.
61 Brat DJ, Lillemoe KD, Yeo CJ, Warfield PB, Hruban RH: Progression of pancreatic intraductal neoplasias to infiltrating adenocarcinoma of the pancreas. Am J Surg Pathol 1998;22: 163–169.
62 Lüttges J, Reinecke-Lüthge A, Möllmann B, Menke MAOH, Clemens A, Klimpfinger M, Sipos B, Klöppel G: Duct changes and k-ras mutations in the disease-free pancreas: analysis of type, age relation and spatial distribution. Virch Arch 1999;435:461–468.
63 Kimura W, Zhao B, Futakawa N, Muto T, Makuuchi M: Significance of k-ras codon 12 point mutation in pancreatic juice in the diagnosis of carcinoma of the pancreas. Hepatogastroenterology 1999;46:532–539.
64 Löhr M, Maisonneuve P, Lowenfels AB: K-ras mutations and benign pancreatic disease. Int J Pancreatol 2000;27:93–103.
65 Luttges J, Diederichs A, Menke MA, Vogel I, Kremer B, Kloppel G: Ductal lesions in patients with chronic pancreatitis show K-ras mutations in a frequency similar to that in the normal pancreas and lack nuclear immunoreactivity for p53. Cancer 2000;88:2495–2504.
66 Guide to Clinical Preventive Services, 2nd Edition, 1996. Report of the U.S. Preventive Services Task Force. Agency for Healthcare Research and Quality, Rockville, MD. http://www.ahrq.gov/clinic/uspstfab.htm.
67 Ulrich CD for the Consensus Committees of the European Registry of Hereditary Pancreatic Diseases, the Midwest Multi-Center Pancreatic Study Group and the International Association of Pancreatology: Pancreatic Cancer in Hereditary Pancreatitis: Consensus Guidelines for Prevention, Screening and Treatment. Pancreatology 2001;1:416–422.

Review Article

Digestive Diseases

Dig Dis 2002;20:38–48

Ulcerative Colitis and Colon Cancer: Strategies for Cancer Prevention

Simon Campbell[a] Subrata Ghosh[b]

[a]Milton Keynes General Hospital, Eaglestone, Milton Keynes, [b]Gastroenterology Section, Imperial College School of Medicine, Hammersmith Hospital, Du Cane Road, London, UK

Key Words
Ulcerative colitis · Colon cancer · Cancer surveillance · Dysplasia

Abstract
The risk of development of colon cancer in patients with ulcerative colitis is an emotive issue with patients and a potential medico-legal problem for physicians caring for such patients. The exact magnitude of the risk is not clearly defined. Current surveillance programmes use dysplasia as a marker for the risk of invasive carcinoma development, but this strategy has inherent limitations. A number of new molecular markers have been investigated but none are currently considered robust enough for routine clinical use. Recommendations for patient selection and interval for colonoscopic surveillance are currently pragmatic, and not entirely evidence-based. Nevertheless, optimal medical management and adherence to a surveillance programme geared to detect dysplasia might still be the best risk reduction strategy.

Introduction

Colorectal carcinoma (CRC), as a complication of ulcerative colitis (UC), was first described as far back as in 1925 by Crohn and Rosenberg [1]. Since then numerous studies have attempted to quantify the degree of increased CRC risk in patients with UC. Studies have reported variable cumulative cancer rates ranging from as little as 1.4% at 18 years [2] to as high as 34% at 25 years [3]. There is general consensus that UC patients at most risk are those with extensive disease and those who have had disease for a duration longer than 8 years [4].

Prior to 1970, prophylactic panproctocolectomy was advocated for UC patients with extensive disease of duration longer than 10 years [5, 6]. Since then, the acccepted model of cancer progression involving dysplasia as a premalignant condition has made surveillance an attractive option in UC patients. Although CRC in UC accounts for only 1% of cases of CRC in the general population [7], CRC may account for upto 17% of all deaths in UC [4] and hence is a population sub-set that would be worthy of a surveillance program.

This article will review the evidence of past and present surveillance strategies that have been published in the literature and present an up-to-date summary of these

KARGER

Fax + 41 61 306 12 34
E-Mail karger@karger.ch
www.karger.com

0257–2753/02/0201–0038$18.50/0

Accessible online at:
www.karger.com/journals/ddi

Prof. Subrata Ghosh
Gastroenterology Section, Imperial College School of Medicine
Hammersmith Hospital, Du Cane Road
London W12 0NN (UK)
Tel. +44 208 8383 1000, E-Mail s.ghosh@ic.ac.uk

findings. Pragmatic strategies for colon cancer prevention and specific problems associated with such preventive strategies for UC sufferers are outlined.

The Risk of Colorectal Carcinoma in Ulcerative Colitis

Despite the risk of CRC in patients with UC being recognized for years, there is considerable controversy over the exact magnitude of this risk. Choi and Kim [8] reviewed published data and calculated the relative risk in UC to vary between 1 and 20 when compared to the general population. The largest epidemiological study to date that analyzed the frequency of CRC in UC examined 3117 Swedish patients between 1922 and 1983 and calculated the relative risk of CRC to be 5.7 in UC versus the general population [9]. This study quantified the relative risk (RR) for CRC in pancolitis (RR = 14.8), left sided disease (RR = 2.8) and proctitis (RR = 1.7), confirming the influence of increasing extent of disease. Finally this study examined the relative risk of CRC according to age at diagnosis, reporting that a younger age at diagnosis carried a significant risk of later CRC. The authors suggested that prophylactic proctocolectomy in patients diagnosed with UC before the age of 15 years may be preferable to close surveillance in reducing mortality in these patients.

Lennard-Jones et al. [10] looked prospectively at 401 UC patients with extensive disease over 22 years. The cumulative probability of developing CRC was 3% at 15 years, 5% at 20 years and 9% at 25 years. Other retrospective studies have assessed cumulative risk of CRC in UC patients with extensive disease to be variable between 34% at 25 years [3] and 1.4% at 18 years [2]. One study in Israel reported even lower risk rates [11] although another study in Israel reported cumulative incidence of CRC in 1035 patients to be 0.2% at 10 years, 2.8% at 15 years and 13.5% at 30 years disease duration [12].

These apparent discrepancies have been put down to differences in follow-up, methods of analysis, differences in study populations (age at diagnosis, geographical location, referral centres), extent of UC at diagnosis and differing colectomy rates in the study groups. Population based estimates provide a much more reliable estimate of the risk than hospital based studies. The reason for apparent differences in cancer risk between world-wide study populations may represent differing interactions between genetic and environmental factors but this remains unclear. Table 1 presents the clinical risk factors associated with an increased CRC risk.

Table 1. Factors influencing risk of colorectal cancer development in ulcerative colitis

Extensive extent of disease
Long duration of disease
Young age at onset
Family history of colorectal cancer
Sclerosing cholangitis
Ongoing chronic inflammatory activity

The only meta-analysis to date has been by Eaden et al. [13] who performed a comprehensive stratified risk analysis – encompassing UC disease anatomy, patient age and geographical location. The estimated risk of CRC in all patients with UC was found to be 2% at 10 years, 8% at 20 years and 18% at 30 years (irrespective of disease extent). They also found that risk of CRC in children was higher than that of adults and that CRC rates were higher in the US and UK compared to Scandinavia and other countries. CRC rates in patients with total colitis were less reliable because of the small numbers in the analysis. Meta-analysis however poses methodological difficulties, as there is considerable heterogeneity amongst the different studies, and approaches to diagnosis and prevention vary widely amongst different centres. The earlier studies have influenced clinical practice considerably, but are different from later studies in optimal medical therapy and diagnostic investigation of choice.

Patients treated with azathioprine or 6-mercaptopurine do not appear to have an increased risk of CRC compared to controls [14,15] although other risk factors for CRC in UC do require further study. Controversy surrounds whether patients with primary sclerosing cholangitis require more rigorous surveillance [16, 17], and whether or not disease modifying medications such as 5-aminosalicylates reduce the necessity for surveillance [18].

Dysplasia as the Endpoint of Surveillance

Progression to CRC in the normal population is thought to proceed through a sequence of genetic and morphological alterations in a pre-cancerous adenomatous polyp. The events preceding CRC in UC are less well defined, but it is thought that dysplastic mucosa precedes CRC (fig. 1). Dysplasia is defined by abnormal crypt architecture (crypts may be irregularly branched, crowded together or reduced in number) and cytological detail

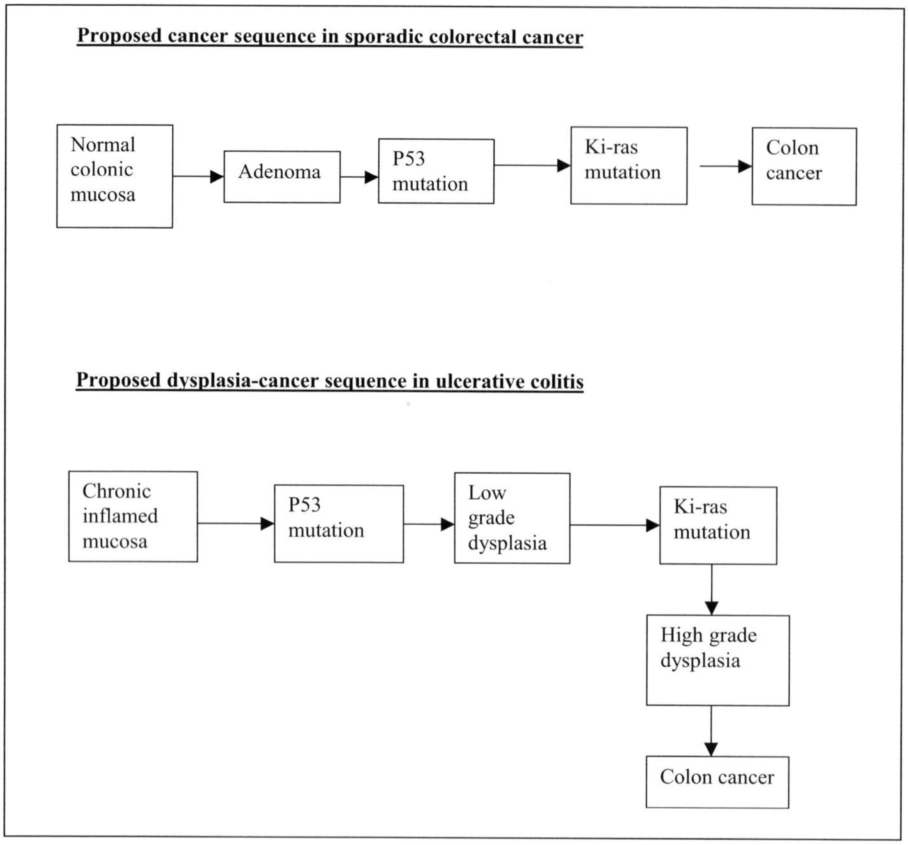

Fig. 1. Sequence of neoplastic transformation to colorectal cancer in sporadic cases and in ulcerative colitis.

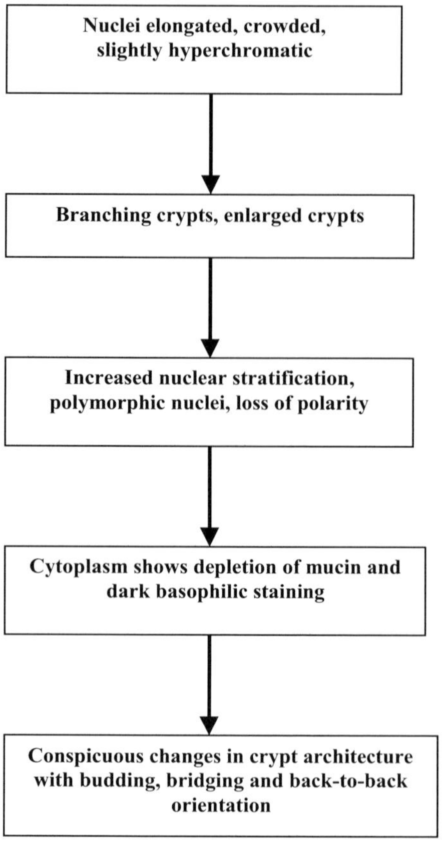

Fig. 2. Morphological progression of dysplasia in ulcerative colitis epithelium.

Table 2. Classification of dysplasia in ulcerative colitis

Negative
Indefinite
Positive
Low-grade
High-grade

The grade of dysplasia is determined by the morphological features of the most dysplastic area of the biopsies.

(nuclei may be pleomorphic or demonstrate hyperchromasia). Morphological progression of dysplasia is illustrated in figure 2. The term dysplasia should only be used for unequivocal, non-invasive neoplastic transformation of the epithelium excluding all reactive changes. Dysplasia of any grade should be regarded as a neoplastic transformation. The currently used categories of dysplasia are shown in table 2. There are well recognized problems using dysplasia as a marker of cancer risk in UC. Dysplasia, despite its classification into low and high grade is a continuum of clonal genetic changes of epithelial cells. It has been shown that there can be considerable interobserver variation even amongst experienced pathologists (4–8%) [19, 20] and presumably this may be higher among non-expert pathologists and in the grading of low-grade dysplasia. In addition, inflammation in colonic mucosa can make the diagnosis of dysplasia even more difficult [19].

The association of dysplasia with cancer in UC is strongest if dysplasia is found in the vicinity of a lesion or mass – a '**D**ysplasia **A**ssociated **L**esion or **M**ass' (DALM) [21]. The chance of a DALM harboring a CRC is as high as upto 40 or 60% depending on the presence of low-grade or high grade dysplasia respectively [21–25], and hence is an indication for colectomy. The presence of dysplasia outwith of a DALM also remains a risk factor for the pres-

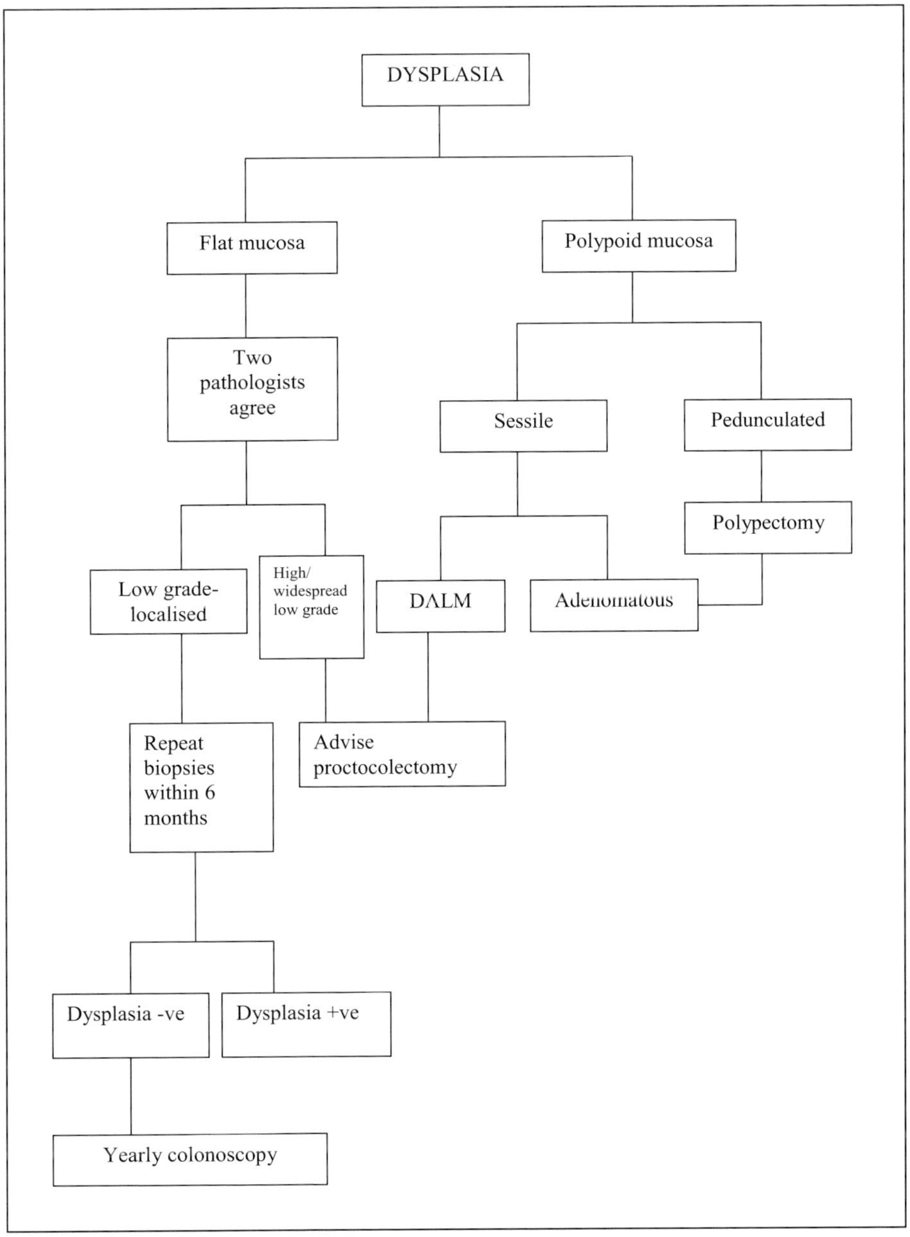

Fig. 3. Clinical decision based on detection of dysplasia in ulcerative colitis.

ence of CRC. Approximately 40% of patients with high grade dysplasia will have a CRC on a subsequent surgical resection specimen [26] – again high-grade dysplasia clearly being an indication for colectomy. The presence of low-grade dysplasia found on biopsy remains a grey area. The prevalence of CRC is lower (3–20%) [25, 27] and there remains differing views as to whether this lesion requires more frequent surveillance or colectomy. One approach is illustrated in figure 3, but more aggressive or more conservative approaches are also advocated. DALM might be difficult to distinguish from a sessile adenomatous polyp, but absence of dysplasia in the epithelium adjacent to the adnomatous polyp is an important distinction.

There have been numerous reports of CRC being diagnosed in patients without dysplasia being detected on previous colonoscopy [23, 28]. Therefore the absence of dysplasia on colonoscopic surveillance does not provide the reassurance about the absence of CRC.

Which Surveillance Strategy?

Prophylactic Colectomy

This remains the definitive strategy in the prevention of the development of CRC in UC patients. As a primary strategy this remains largely unacceptable to both physicians and patients, since there are considerable social and medical drawbacks of an ileostomy or ileal-pouch anal anastomosis. There is no published data that helps shed light on patient preferences or patients' quality of life as compared to those who undergo a surveillance program. It should be remembered that well over 80% of UC patients do not eventually develop CRC! However, the topic is emotive and fear of cancer is one of the prime concerns of patients with UC.

Colonoscopic Surveillance

This is the most widely practised strategy, and has been shown to be a relatively safe procedure [29]. The ultimate goal of mortality reduction is by detecting pre-cancerous dysplastic lesions in the colon or at least earlier CRC in UC patients. It should be noted that the average colon (approximately 1 metre in length) has a total surface area of 1.2 m^2, and 10 surveillance biopsies would cover a surface area of approximately 60 mm^2 (less then 0.05% of the total surface area). There has been considerable speculation as to the impact of such sampling on detecting dysplasia and subsequently its impact on mortality reduction. A reasonable sampling strategy is to obtain at least 2 biopsies at 10-cm intervals throughout the colon as well as biopsies from any suspicious areas. In addition, there have been a large number of studies looking at the effects of colonoscopy on these goals, but several studies have included small patient groups of less than 100 patients [30, 31]. Analysis of colonoscopic screening practice in the UK has been shown to be disorganized. In one study of UK practice, only 45% of colonoscopic biopsies were reviewed by a specialist in gastroenterology pathology and only 53% of gastroenterologists recommended colectomy after dysplasia was detected by colonoscopy [32]. Surveys of American gastroenterologists were similar. The St. Marks' experience is probably the most quoted study to date, and the first to publish extensive prospective data on a large number of UC patients who had undergone colonoscopic surveillance [33] (sigmoidoscopy was used in the initial part of their study, since colonoscopy was not available till 1970). This study looked at 303 patients (186 had UC for 10 years or more) between 1966 and 1980 and detected 8 patients with dysplasia. The study reported a significant number of patients who developed cancer during surveillance (n = 13), and 11 of these were deemed potentially curable (Dukes A-C). The study recommended consideration of colectomy in patients with UC beyond 10 years or very careful follow-up in these patients. Rosenstock et al. [20] published their retrospective experience on 248 patients in 1985. Mean disease duration was 12 years at the time of inclusion. This group was particularly heterogenous – 24% had disease of less than 8 years, 69% had only one colonoscopic examination, while 31% had more than one colonoscopy (mean interval of 19 months between colonoscopies). They found an overall incidence of high-grade dysplasia of 6% (n = 15), and found CRC in 3% (n = 7). This study concluded that dysplasia was a reliable histopathological marker and correlated with CRC in chronic UC, supporting the use of surveillance colonoscopy. Nugent et al. [24] performed 2 yearly colonoscopic surveillances in 213 patients over a 13-year period. Mean duration of disease was 14 years (range 8–39 years), median duration of histological follow-up was 4 years and on average 19 biopsies were taken at each colonoscopy. Six patients died of CRC in this study (4 were initially diagnosed with dysplasia and underwent colectomy at that stage, 2 were negative for dysplasia). The 2 patients who were negative for dysplasia had inadequate surveillance, while another 4 patients who were diagnosed with dysplasia were cured by colectomy. These findings suggested that negative biopsies for dysplasia was a predictor of being free of CRC, albeit tempered by the fact they did not have a control group of chronic UC patients who were not undergoing surveillance. In addition, the risk of CRC in pan-colitis was found in this cohort to be the same as that of patients with left-sided disease. These results supported the use of such a surveillance program. Lindberg et al. [34] published their 20-year prospective study of 143 patients with extensive disease of more than 10 years duration. Two-yearly colonoscopies were performed on these patients. Double biopsies were taken from 9 locations on each colonoscopy, and detected 48 (34%) patients with dysplasia (cured by colectomy) and 7 (4%) CRCs, of which only 2 patients were cured by colectomy – 5 patients diagnosed with CRC died. Of note in this study was that the predictive value of low-grade and high-grade dysplasia for CRC was particularly low at 14%. Although they concluded that colonoscopic surveillance might have a role in reducing mortality, they advocated the possible use of complementary histopathological markers such as DNA aneuploidy.

Finally, Karlen et al. [35] addressed the goal of this type of surveillance – mortality. This retrospective analysis examined all UC patients who died from CRC who had undergone surveillance colonoscopy (n = 42) and compared them with matched controls (n = 102, matched for disease extent, disease duration, age and sex). They found a trend toward a protective effect of colonoscopic surveillance against death, but this did not reach statistical significance. This study was limited somewhat however by its retrospective design, lack of data available from case records, and that the patient database was taken from the 1970's – a time when surveillance was done less commonly and when histological definitions for dysplasia were different to what is current practice. Others have tried to draw conclusions on the impact on mortality by using mathematical models of hypothetical cohorts of UC patients. Recently, Delco and Sonnenberg [36] used the Markov model and compared cost-benefit outcomes in patients undergoing and those not undergoing a surveillance program. Albeit that such models make strict assumptions that may not be easily extrapolated into real-world populations, this modelling analysis did not find it possible to prove that colonoscopic surveillance was an effective means to manage the increased risk of CRC in UC patients.

DNA Aneuploidy – Flow Cytometric Analysis

In light of the inter-observer variation associated with dysplasia classification and furthermore of the uncertainty that surrounds the natural progression of dysplasia in UC patients, there has been numerous searches to obtain a more sensitive and specific marker of pre-malignancy. The candidate molecular markers are presented in table 4. Flow cytometry is used to detect deoxyribonucleic acid (DNA) aneuploidy from colonic biopsies taken at colonoscopy. DNA aneuploidy (DNAa) has been shown to be absent in normal colonic mucosa and present in up to 70% of CRCs [37–42]. The presence of DNAa in colonic mucosa of patient with UC was first described in 1984 in a patient who, a year later, developed a CRC in the same anatomical area [43]. Since then, further reports have confirmed the presence of DNAa in conjunction with histopathologically defined dysplasia [44, 45]. The significance of DNAa without dysplasia remains unclear [46]. Melville et al. [47] looked at 333 paraffin blocks from 58 UC patients with extensive, chronic disease (22 had developed CRC), and correlated DNAa with dysplasia and CRC. They concluded that DNAa was easier to recognize than dysplasia, correlated with dysplasia and CRC, and that it was a useful marker of pre-malignant disease in UC. This study advocated its use to complement histologic examination when dysplasia is suspected. Rutegard et al. reported their experience with DNAa in UC patients [48]. In this study flow cytometry was performed on 25 patients with dysplasia (indeterminate dysplasia n = 11, low grade dysplasia n = 11, high grade dysplasia n = 3). Two patients who developed CRC were excluded from the study. Six patients (19 biopsies) with DNAa were finally examined. Of these, 14 biopsies out of 19 (74%) had definite or indefinite histological dysplasia. Although these results supported an association between dysplasia and DNAa, these results highlight thefact that the two do not constantly co-exist. Importantly, one patient who developed CRC did so without any evidence of dysplasia. Prospective data has been published by Lofberg et al. [45]. Fifty-nine patients with longstanding, extensive UC were followed up in a colonoscopic surveillance program. These patients had UC for at least 8 years (median disease duration 21 years, range 11–45 years) and patients underwent 2-yearly colonoscopy. Twenty biopsies were taken from 10 predetermined areas. A total of 916 DNA samples were evaluated (only 6 were not possible to analyse). Fifteen of the 59 patients had demonstrable DNAa at least once, and findings of DNAa were distributed evenly and randomly throughout the colon. DNAa was detected in 6 patients before dysplasia had developed by an average of 2.7 years. The remaining other 6 patients in whom DNAa was demonstrated also had concomitant dysplasia. In summary, this provided further evidence that DNAa probably precedes dysplasia. However, the study concluded that more information and answers were required about what to do in patients with DNAa without dysplasia, in whom repeat biopsies are negative, before flow cytometry analysis could be used as a replacement for dysplasia surveillance. Flow cytometry is not susceptible to significant inter-observer variation compared with detection of dysplasia.

Other questions with regard DNAa remain. In animal models, DNAa has been shown to disappear if the causing carcinogenetic influence is removed [49] – and it remains to be proved whether this is true in humans, and indeed whether a repeated negative biopsy for DNAa is reassuring or not. The use of flow cytometry and DNAa analysis remains an adjunct and not a replacement for dysplasia surveillance.

p53 and Ki Ras Expression

Significant differences exist between the development of CRC in UC when compared to sporadic CRC. Although both DNAa and loss of the p53 tumour suppressor allele are often found in adenocarcinoma in both situations [50–52], there remains significant differences. Studies by Burmer et al. [50] have suggested that loss of heterozygosity for the p53 (p53 LOH) allele may occur earlier in the neoplastic progression in UC when compared to sporadic CRC where it is seen as a later event in the adenoma to cancer transition (fig. 1). This group later examined DNAa and p53 LOH in 9 UC patients with extensive, chronic disease(>10 years) [51]. These 9 patients consisted of 3 with CRC, 5 with high grade dysplasia, and 1 with low grade dysplasia were analysed by flow-cytometry. The presence of p53 LOH was found in 22/26 biopsies in the CRC group, 25/40 in the high-grade dysplasia group and 7/21 biopsy specimens with LGD. They concluded that DNAa was an earlier event than p53 LOH, but the latter was a more specific marker for the presence of dysplasia or CRC in a biopsy. In addition, these changes were often found in histologically normal (i.e. non-dysplastic) areas of the colon, suggesting that such changes are a field change within the colon of patients with UC. Lashner et al. [53] has further evaluated the usefulness of p53 LOH by immunohistochemical staining techniques. They examined a cohort of 95 patients with longstanding pancolitis who were in a surveillance program. In this study, the presence of p53 gave a relative risk of 4.53 (CI 2.16–9.48) of developing dysplasia and preceded the presence of high grade dysplasia and CRC by 26 months and 38 months respectively. Interestingly, they found that folic acid supplementation had a small but significant protective effect for p53 mutations (relative risk 0.97, CI 0.94–1.00).

Ki-Ras is a proto-oncogene, and mutations of Ki-Ras have been shown to be present in up to 60% of all sporadic CRCs [54, 55]. A slightly lower frequency of this mutation has been noted in CRCs present in longstanding UC [56]. Studies to date point to the occurrence of Ki-Ras mutations in colonic mucosa later than p53 mutations [57]. Wong et al. [58] looked at immunohistochemical techniques to evaluate Ki67 and p53 expression in the assessment of UC-related dysplasia. This detailed study examined 70 pathology sections from 44 cases of UC (regenerative atypia n = 22, low grade dysplasia n = 22, high grade dysplasia n = 14, indefinite for dysplasia n = 12). They found inter-observer and intra-observer reproducibility in scoring Ki67 and p53 variation to be good; the negative predictive value of p53 staining was 73% excluding a diagnosis of HGD, this was in comparison to 36% for Ki67. The two tests combined gave a negative predictive value of 83%. Despite the low predictive value of Ki67 shown in this study, it was noted that restriction of Ki67 immuno-staining to the basal third of the crypt excluded the diagnosis of dysplasia. Holzmann et al. [57] confirmed this data using 1486 biopsies from 83 patients. They compared p53, Ki-ras mutations with DNAa and found strong correlation coefficients for dysplasia and DNAa ($p < 0.001$), dysplasia and p53 ($p = 0.05$) and between dysplasia and p53 and/or Ki-ras mutations ($p = 0.002$). No significant associations were found with Ki-ras mutations alone. Other studies have also confirmed the reproducibility of these findings by PCR analysis on lavage fluid obtained at surveillance colonoscopy [55, 59] which opens the door to other potential methods for obtaining evaluable material for analysis.

Sialosyl-Tn Antigen

Mucin-associated carbohydrates have been shown before to be over-expressed antigens in CRC [60]. Sialosyl-Tn antigen (STn) is a blood group derived antigen that is expressed in up to 90% of CRCs [61, 62] and stainable with TKH2 monoclonal antibody. Although it has yet to be shown that STn expression mirrors the adenoma to CRC sequence in sporadic colon cancer, there is relatively little known in the UC patient model. One study by Itzkowitz et al. [63] examined STn expression in archival tissues from 7 UC patients who developed CRC and 8 controls that did not by immuno-histochemical techniques. They also examined anatomical distribution of STn expression within the colon of resected specimens (n = 17) and controls (n = 6). They found that 86% of the 7 patients had STn expression, whereas 38% of the controls had STn expression. In the other part of the study they found that in cancer bearing colons, 40/82 specimens were STn positive compared with 13% of controls. In particular, STn expression was found in association with high grade dysplasia. This confirmed that STn expression is potentially exciting as a marker of dysplasia as found by others where STn expression occurs in up to 80% of patients with high-grade dysplasia [64]. The same group later performed a more extensive retrospective study examining STn expression in 969 biopsy specimens from UC patients within a surveillance program [65]. They looked at STn expresssion with time and by anatomical location within the colon. Their results demonstrated that STn expression was present throughout the colon and consistent on consecutive biopsies (91%), either preceding dysplasia by up to 7 years or present at the time of histological dysplasia. This adds further strength to STn expression as a useful marker in detecting UC patients at risk of dysplasia. A large prospective study is now required to confirm these results, although a study of 22 UC patients (1691 biopsy specimens) found 47% of patients expressed STn who were referred for colectomy for dysplasia compared to 7% of patients referred because of dis-

Table 3. Proposed molecular markers indicative of neoplastic transformation in ulcerative colitis. None are reliable enough to be used currently for clinical decision making

DNA aneuploidy by flow cytometry
Sialosyl-Tn antigen
P53 mutation or loss of heterozygosity
K-ras mutation
Microsatellite instability
Increased CD44v6 expression in crypts
β-Catenin expression
Chromosomal gain and loss by fluorescent in-situ hybridization (FISH)
Loss of E-cadherin and over-expression of P-cadherin
Loss of heterozygosity for p16
Activation of *src* proto-oncogene
P-glycoprotein overexpression
Laminin-5 gamma 2 chain expression
Cyclin A expression
Proliferating cell nuclear antigen (PCNA)

Table 4. Well recognized problems of surveillance strategy in colorectal carcinoma

Inter-observation variability in dysplasia diagnosis and grading
Difficulty in recognizing DALM amidst irregular mucosa with pseudopolyps
Difficulty in distinguising DALM from adenomatous polyps
Difficulty in determining onset of colitis in patients with PSC
Extension of distal or left sided colitis without change in symptoms
Categorization of extent in patients with localized cecal inflammation in left sided colitis

DALM = Dysplasia-associated lesion or mass.

ease intractability [66]. In addition, STn expression was found to be independent of DNAa (where STn was expressed earlier) as a marker of dysplasia. Table 3 summarizes the various molecular markers which show promise as early markers of neoplastic transformation.

Discussion

It remains undisputed that chronic (>8–10 years duration), extensive UC carries a significant risk of CRC development. However, this risk is difficult to quantify exactly. This is because of uncertainty over the exact duration of disease in particular patients (especially in primary sclerosing cholangitis subgroup), differences in concomitant drug therapy (especially 5-ASA therapy, which may afford protective benefit as suggest by some [67]), changes of disease anatomy with time, differing colectomy rates from centre to centre and possibly geographical location.

Surveillance for CRC in UC would be simplified if the exact model for CRC in UC was known. To date, the basis of CRC surveillance for UC patients is largely based upon current surveillance programs in use for sporadic CRC but there remains significant differences in the pathogenesis in of CRC in UC patients that still remain to be elucidated. Figure 1 shows the currently proposed pathogenesis of CRC in UC compared to sporadic CRC. Leading from this, colonoscopy remains the investigative tool by which surveillance is currently conducted. This has significant drawbacks as mentioned earlier, not to mention the real-world problems of compliance itself – something that would probably have more impact on its relative effectiveness. A summary of the problems inherent in colonoscopic surveillance is presented in table 4. Although 2-yearly surveillance is used by many, the optimal colonscopic surveillance interval remains to be shown. Current recommendations by expert panels are therefore generally pragmatic rather than evidence based (table 5). Evidence from controlled trials, i.e. surveillance vs no surveillance will probably never be available for more definitive guidelines.

Finally the drawbacks of dysplasia classification are plain to see (table 4). Histopathology remains the one modality that has clearly evolved in recent years. A strategy to prevent colorectal cancer is illustrated in figure 4. It is just as important to involve the patient in all decision making, have a multidisciplinary team to counsel patients, have a well organised computerised patient follow-up system and have motivated pathologists and colonoscopists. While high grade dysplasia remains an indication for curative colectomy, the search continues for a more objective and reproducable technique of pre-cancerous lesions. DNAa is probably the most validated technique for looking at pre-dysplastic lesions and is promising. Furthermore, p53 staining and possibly the advent of STn immunostaining are new and exciting techniques for improving selection of patients for curative therapy, but these require further prospective studies before they are applied to clinical surveillance. Perhaps a combination of techniques such as presence of DNAa and STn antigen may improve current criteria for recommending elective colectomy – time will tell ...

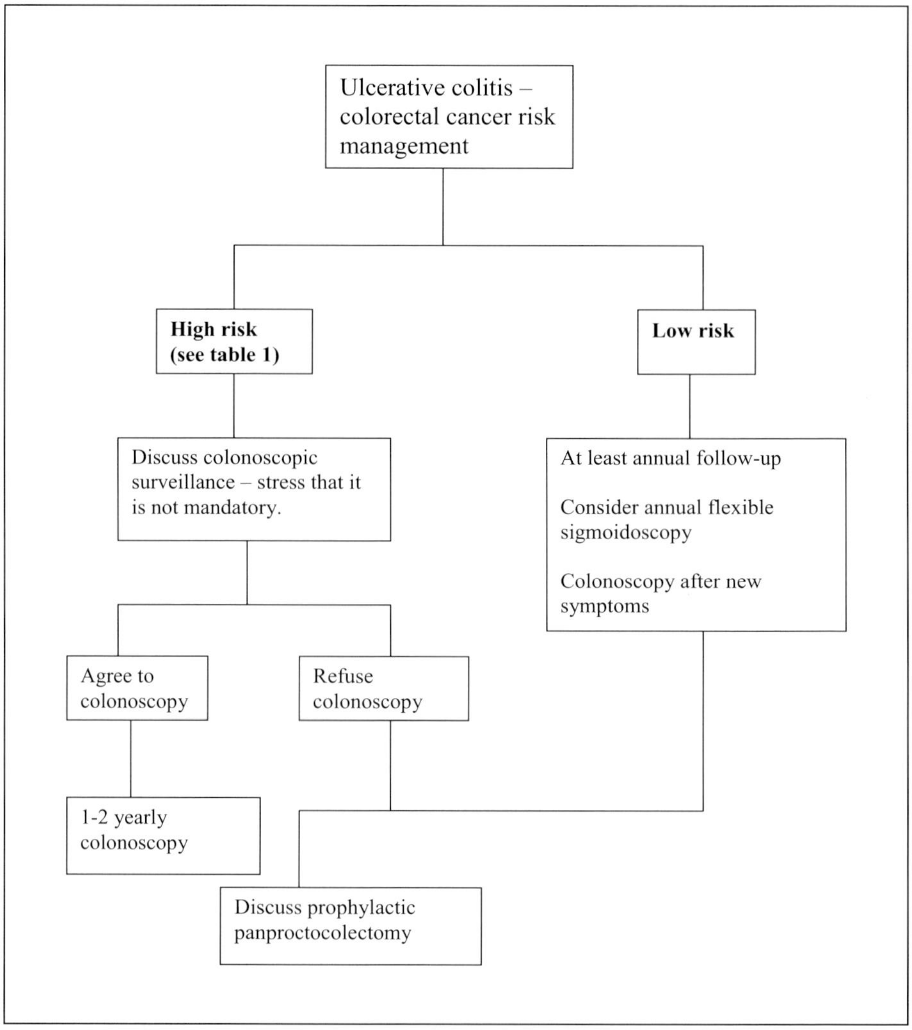

Fig. 4. A strategy for prevention of colorectal cancer in ulcerative colitis patients.

Table 5. Recommendations based on graded evidence for surveillance strategies to prevent colorectal cancer in ulcerative colitis

Recommending authority	Key recommendations
American Gastroenterological Association (AGA) 1997*	Surveillance colonoscopy should be considered in patients with long-standing, extensive inflammatory bowel disease to look for dysplasia Common practice: Surveillance colonoscopy every 1-2 years after 8 years of pancolitis or after 15 years of left-sided colitis
Scottish Intercollegiate Guidelines Network (SIGN) 1997**	Available evidence did not warrant recommendations for cancer screening in inflammatory bowel disease In young patients <45 years old with long-standing inflammatory bowel disease colorectal symptoms should prompt urgent referral and investigation

* Also endorsed by American College of Gastroenterology, Crohn's and Colitis Foundation of America, American Cancer Society, American Society for Gastrointestinal Endoscopy, American Society of Colon and Rectal Surgeons.

** Also endorsed by Scottish Cancer Therapy Network.

References

1 Crohn B, Rosenberg H: The sigmoidoscopic picture of chronic ulcerative colitis (non-specific). Amer J Med Sci 1925;170:220–228.
2 Hendrikson C, Kreiner S, Binder V: Long term prognosis in ulcerative colitis – based on results from a regional patient group from the county of Copenhagen. Gut 1985;26:158–163.
3 Kewenter J, Ahlman H, Hulten L: Cancer risk in extensive ulcerative colitis. Annals of Surg 1978;188:824–828.
4 Gyde S, Prior P, Dew NJ: Mortality in ulcerative colitis. Gastroenterology 1982;83:36–43.
5 de Dombal FT, Watts JM, Watkinson G, Goligher JC: Local complications of ulcerative colitis: Stricture, pseudo-polyposis, and carcinoma of colon and rectum. Brit Med J 1966; ii:1442–1447.
6 Devroede GJ, Taylor WF, Sauer WG, Jackman RJ, Stickler GB: Cancer risk and life expectancy of children with ulcerative colitis. N Engl J Med 1971;285:17–21.
7 Choi P, Zelig MP: Similarity of colorectal cancer in Crohn's disease and ulcerative colitis: Implications for carcinogenesis and prevention. Gut 1994;35:950–954.
8 Choi PM, Kim W: Colon cancer surveillance. Gastroenterol Clin North Am 1995;24:671–687.
9 Ekbom A, Helmick C, Zack M, Adami H-O: Ulcerative colitis and colorectal cancer: A population-based study. N Engl J Med 1990;323: 1228–1233.
10 Lennard-Jones JE, Melville DM, Morson BC, Ritchie JK, Williams CB: Precancer and cancer in extensive ulcerative colitis: Findings among 401 patients over 22 years. Gut 1990;31:800–806.
11 Gilat T, Zemishlany Z, Ribak J, Benaroya Y, Lilos P: Ulcerative colitis in the Jewish population of Tel-Aviv Yafo. Gastroenterology 1974; 67:933–938.
12 Gilat T, Fireman Z, Grossman A, Hacohen D, Kadish U, Ron E, Rozen P, Lilos P: Colorectal cancer in patients with ulcerative colitis. A population study in central Israel. Gastroenterology 1988;94:870–877.
13 Eaden JA, Abrams KR, Mayberry JF: The risk of colorectal cancer in ulcerative colitis: A meta-analysis. Gut 1901;48:526–535.
14 Connell WR, Kamm MA, Dickson M, Balkwill AM, Ritchie JK, Lennard-Jones JE: Long-term neoplasia risk after azathioprine treatment in inflammatory bowel disease. Lancet 1994;343: 1249–1252.
15 Peppercorn MA: 6-mercaptopurine for management of ulcerative colitis: A concept whose time has come. Am J Gastroenterol 1996;91: 1689–1690.
16 Choi PM, Nugent FW, Rossi RL: Relationship between colorectal neoplasia and primary sclerosing cholangitis in ulcerative colitis. Gastroenterology 1992;103:1707–1709.
17 D'Haens GR, Lashner BA, Hanauer SB: Pericholangitis and sclerosing cholangitis are risk factors for dysplasia and cancer in ulcerative colitis. Am J Gastroenterol 1993;88:1174–1178.
18 Pinczowski D, Ekbom A, Baron J, Yuen J, Adami HO: Risk factors for colorectal cancer in patients with ulcerative colitis: A case-control study. Gastroenterology 1994;107:117–120.
19 Butt JH, Price A, Williams CB: Dysplasia and cancer in ulcerative colitis; in Allan RN, Norman R (eds): Inflammatory Bowel Diseases. Edinburgh, Churchill Livingstone, 1983, pp140–153.
20 Rosenstock E, Farmer RG, Petras R: Surveillance for colonic carcinoma in ulcerative colitis. Gastroenterology 1985;89:1342–1346.
21 Blackstone MO, Riddell RH, Rogers BH, Levin B: Dysplasia-associated lesion or mass (DALM) detected by colonscopy in long-standing ulcerative colitis: An indication for colectomy. Gastroenterology 1981;80:366–374.
22 Axon AT: Cancer surveillance in ulcerative colitis: A time for reappraisal. Gut 1994;35:587–589.
23 Bernstein CN, Shanahan F, Weinstein WM: Are we telling patients the truth about surveillance colonoscopy in ulcerative colitis? Lancet 1994;343:71–74.
24 Nugent FW, Haggitt RC, Gilpin PA: Cancer surveillance in ulcerative colitis. Gastroenterology 1991;100:1241–1248.
25 Woolrich AJ, DaSilva MD, Korelitz BI: Surveillance in the routine management of ulcerative colitis: The predictive value of low-grade dysplasia. Gastroenterology 1992;103:431–438.
26 Ransohoff DF, Riddell RH, Levin B: Ulcerative colitis and cancer: Problems in assessing the diagnostic usefulness of mucosal dysplasia. Dis Colon Rectum 1985;28:383–388.
27 Rubin CE, Haggit RC, Burmer GC, Brentwall TA, Stevens AC, Levine DS, Dean PJ, Kimmey M, Perera DR, Rabinovitch PS: DNA aneuploidy in colonic biopsies predicts future development. Gastroenterology 1992;103:1611–1620.
28 Collins JR, Feldman M, Fordtran JS: Colon cancer, dysplasia, and surveillance in patients with ulcerative colitis. A critical review. N Engl J Med 1987;316:1654–1658.
29 Koobatian GJ, Choi PM: Safety of surveillance colonoscopy in long-standing ulcerative colitis. Am J Gastroenterol 1994;89:1472–1475.
30 Brostrom O, Lofberg R, Ost A, Reichard H: Cancer surveillance of patients with longstanding ulcerative colitis: A clinical, endoscopical, and histological study. Gut 1986;27:1408–1413.
31 Choi PM, Nugent FW, Schoetz JD, Silverman ML, Haggitt RC: Colonoscopic surveillance reduces mortality from colorectal cancer in ulcerative colitis. Gastroenterology 1993;105:418–424.
32 Eaden JA, Ward BA, Mayberry JF: How gastroenterologists screen for colonic cancer in ulcerative colitis: An analysis of performance. Gastrointest Endosc 2000;51:123–128.
33 Lennard-Jones JE, Morson BC, Ritchie JK: Cancer surveillance in ulcerative colitis. Lancet 1983;ii:149–152.
34 Lindberg B, Persson B, Veress B, Ingelman-Sundberg H, Granqvist S: Twenty years' colonoscopic surveillance of patients with ulcerative colitis. Detection of dysplastic and malignant transformation. Scand J Gastroenterol 1996; 31:1195–1204.
35 Karlen P, Kornfeld D, Brostrom O, Lofberg R, Persson P-G, Ekbom A: Is colonoscopic surveillance reducing colorectal cancer mortality in ulcerative colitis? A population based case control study. Gut 1998;42:711–714.
36 Delco F, Sonnenberg A: A decision analysis of surveillance for colorectal cancer in ulcerative colitis. Gut 2000;46:500–506.
37 Armitage N, Robins RA, Evans DF, Turner DR, Baldwin RW, Hardcastle JD: The influence of tumour cell DNA abnormailities on survival in colorectal cancer. Brit J Surg 1985; 72:828–830.
38 Banner BF, Tomas-de la Vega JE, Roseman DL, Coon JS: Should flow cytometric DNA analysis precede definitive surgery for colon carcinoma? Ann Surg 1985;202:740–744.
39 Kokal W, Scheibani K, Terz J, Harada R: Tumour DNA content in the prognosis of colorectal carcinoma. JAMA 1986;255:3123–3127.
40 Melamed MR, Enker WE, Banner P, Janov AJ, Kessler G, Darzynkiewicz Z: Flow cytometry of colorectal carcinoma with three-year follow-up. Dis Colon Rectum 1986;29:184–186.
41 Tribukait B, Hammarberg C, Rubio C: Ploidy and proliferation patterns in colorectal adenocarcinomas related to Dukes' classification and to histopathological differentiation. Acta Pathol Microbiol Immunol Scand 1983;91:89–95.
42 Wolley RC, Schreiber K, Koss LG, Karas M, Sherman A: DNA distribution in human colon carcinomas and its relationship to clinical behaviour. JNCI 1982;69:15–22.
43 Hammarberg C, Slezak P, Tribukait B: Flow cytometric DNA analysis as a means for early detection of malignancy in patients with chronic ulcerative colitis. Gut 1984;25:905–908.
44 Hammarberg C, Slezak P, Tribukait B: Early detection of malignancy in ulcerative colitis: a flow cytometric study. Cancer 1984;53:291–295.
45 Lofberg R, Brostrom O, Karlen P, Ost A, Tribukait B: DNA aneuploidy in ulcerative colitis: Reproducibility, topographic distribution, and relation to dysplasia. Gastroenterology 1992; 102:1149–1154.
46 Fozard JBJ, Quirke P, Dixon MF, Giles GR, Bird CC: DNA aneuploidy in ulcerative colitis. Gut 1986;27:1414–1418.

47 Melville DM, Jass JR, Shepherd NA, Northover JMA, Capellaro D, Richman PI, Lennard-Jones JE, Ritchie JK, Andersen SN: Dysplasia and deoxyribonucleic acid aneuploidy in the assessment of precancerous changes in chronic ulcerative colitis. Observer variation and correlations. Gastroenterology 1988;95:668–675.
48 Rutegard J, Ahsgren L, Stenling R, Roos G: DNA content in ulcerative colitis. Flow cytometric analysis in a patient series from a defined area. Dis Colon Rectum 1988;31:710–715.
49 Auer G, Ono J, Nasiell M, Caspersson T: Reversibility of bronchial cell atypia. Cancer Res 1982;42:4241–4247.
50 Burmer GC, Crispin DA, Kolli VR, Haggitt RC, Kulander BG, Rubin CE, Rabinovitch PR: Frequent loss of a p53 allele in carcinomas and their precursors in Ulcerative Colitis. Cancer Commun 1991;3:167–172.
51 Burmer GC, Rabinovitch PS, Haggitt RC, Crispin DA, Brentnall TA, Kolli VR, Stevens AC, Rubin CE: Neoplastic progression in ulcerative colitis: Histology, DNA content, and loss of a p53 allele. Gastroenterology 1992;103:1602–1610.
52 Riddell RH, Goldman H, Ransohoff DF, Appelman HD, Fenoglio CM, Haggitt RC, Ahren C, Correa P, Hamilton SR, Morson BC, et al: Dysplasia in inflammatory bowel: standardized classification with provisional clinical applications. Hum Pathol 1983;14:931–968.
53 Lashner BA, Shapiro BD, Husain A, Goldblum JR: Evaluation of the usefulness of testing for p53 mutations in colorectal cancer surveillance for ulcerative colitis. Am J Gastroenterol 1999;94:456–462.
54 Holzman K, Klump B, Borchard F, Hsieh C-J, Kuhn A, Gaco V, Gregor M, Porschen R: Comparative analysis of histology, DNA content, p53 and Ki-ras mutations in colectomy specimens with long-standing ulcerative colitis. Int J Cancer 1998;76:1–6.
55 Lang SM, Heinzlmann M, Stratakis DF, Teschauer W, Loeschke K: Detection of Ki-ras mutations by PCR and differential hybridization and of p53 mutations by SSCP analysis in endoscopically obtained lavage solution from patients with long-standing ulcerative colitis. Am J Gastroenterol 1997;92:2166–2170.
56 Burmer GC, Levine DS, Kulander BG, Haggitt RC, Rubin CE, Rabinovitch PS: c-Ki-ras mutations in chronic ulcerative colitis and sporadic colon carcinoma. Gastroenterology 1990;50:7717–7722.
57 Holzmann K, Weis-Klemm M, Klump B, Hsieh C-J, Borchard F, Gregor M, Porschen R: Comparison of flow cytometry and histology with mutational screening for p53 and Ki-ras mutations in surveillance of patients with long-standing ulcerative colitis. Scand J Gastroenterol 2001;36:1320–1326.
58 Wong NACS, Mayer NJ, MacKell S, Gilmour HM, Harrison DJ: Immunohistochemical assessment of Ki67 and p53 expression assists the diagnosis and grading of ulcerative colitis-related dysplasia. Histopathology 2000;37:108–114.
59 Lang SM, Stratakis DF, Heinzlmann M, Heldwein W, Wiebecke B, Loeschke K: Molecular screening of patients with long standing extensive ulcerative colitis: Detection of p53 and Ki-ras mutations by single strand conformation polymorphism analysis and differential hybridisation in colonic lavage fluid. Gut 1999;44:822–825.
60 Itzkowitz S: Carbohydrate changes in colon carcinoma. APMIS 1992;100:173–180.
61 Itzkowitz S, Yuan M, Montgomery CK, Kjeldsen T, Takahashi HK, Bigbee WL, Kim YS: Expresssion of Tn, sialosyl Tn, and T antigens in human colon cancer. Cancer Res 1989;49:197–204.
62 Itzkowitz SH, Bloom EJ, Kokal WA, Modin G, Hakomori S, Kim YS: Sialosyl-Tn: A novel mucin antigen associated with prognosis in colorectal cancer patients. Cancer 1990;66:1960–1966.
63 Itzkowitz SH, Marshall A, Kornbluth A, Harpaz N, McHugh JBD, Ahnen D, Sachar DB: Sialosyl-Tn antigen: Initial report of a new marker of malignant progression in long-standing ulcerative colitis. Gastroenterology 1995;109:490–497.
64 Thor A, Itzkowitz SH, Schlom J, Kim YS, Hanauer SB: Tumor-associated glycoprotein (TAG-72) expresssion in ulcerative colitis. Int J Cancer 1989;43:810–815.
65 Itzkowitz SH, Young E, Dubois D, Harpaz N, Bodian C, Chen A, Sachar DB: Sialosyl-Tn antigen is prevalent and precedes dysplasia in ulcerative colitis: A retrospective case-control study. Gastroenterology 1996;110:694–704.
66 Karlen P, Young E, Brostrom O, Lofberg R, Tribukait B, Ost A, Bodian C, Itzkowitz S: Sialyl-Tn antigen as a marker of colon cancer risk in ulcerative colitis: Relation to dysplasia and DNA aneuploidy. Gastroenterology 1998;115:1395–1404.
67 Eaden J, Abrams K, Ekbom A, Jackson E, Mayberry J: Colorectal cancer prevention in ulcerative colitis: A case-control study. Aliment Pharmacol Ther 2000;14:145–153.

Review Article

Digestive Diseases

Dig Dis 2002;20:49–60

Neuroendocrine Tumors of the Gastro-Entero-Pancreatic System: The Role of Early Diagnosis, Genetic Testing and Preventive Surgery

U. Plöckinger B. Wiedenmann

Medizinische Klinik m. S. Hepatologie, Gastroenterologie, Endokrinologie und Stoffwechsel, Charité, Campus Virchow-Klinikum, Humboldt Universität zu Berlin, Germany

Key Words

Neuroendocrine tumors · Gastroenteropancreatic system · Diagnosis · Therapy

Abstract

Surgery is the only curative approach in neuroendocrine gastro-entero-pancreatic (GEP) tumors. As cure is highly dependent of tumor size, early diagnosis is a prerequisite for surgical success. Diagnosis of nonfunctioning tumors of the pancreas or midgut origin is due to symptoms related to the tumor burden, thus early diagnosis is mostly incidental. Functioning pancreatic tumors should be operated early in the course of the disease to provide cure. No genetic screening is available for sporadic GEP tumors. In patients with MEN-1 syndrome genetic screening is recommended to restrict the burden of clinical screening to those with positive test results. Due to the nature of the disease cure may not be achieved, however prevention of cancer may be obtained for one or two decades of life, especially in patients with gastrinoma or nonfunctioning tumors.

Introduction

Neuroendocrine tumors of the gastro-entero-pancreatic (GEP) system are rare, with an incidence of 1–2/100,000/year equally distributed between the sexes [1]. Early diagnosis is mandatory, as the cure rate in sporadic tumors is highly dependent on tumor size. Timely diagnosis should be facilitated by a broad knowledge of signs and symptoms characteristic for these tumors, the use of adequate diagnostic tools and correct interpretation of test results. The focus of this review is on epidemiological, clinical and diagnostic data in sporadic functioning and nonfunctioning tumors of the pancreas and midgut. In addition, these tumors are discussed as part of the multiple endocrine neoplasia syndrome type-1 (MEN-1).

Classification

The classification of GEP tumors as functional/nonfunctional is based on symptoms due to hypersecretion of hormones, neuropeptides or neurotransmitters. Nonfunctioning tumors are neoplasms of neuroendocrine differentiation without symptoms due to hormonal hypersecretion. However, these tumors may have immuno-histochemically detectable hormone production. Hormone secretion may be defective or occur at a low, subclinical level. Secreted hormones may be clinically ineffective or a defective hormone synthesis may produce

KARGER

Fax + 41 61 306 12 34
E-Mail karger@karger.ch
www.karger.com

0257–2753/02/0201–0049$18.50/0

Accessible online at:
www.karger.com/journals/ddi

Prof. Dr. B. Wiedenmann, Humboldt Universität zu Berlin, Charité
Campus Virchow-Klinikum, Medizinische Klinik m. S. Hepatologie, Gastroenterologie, Endokrinologie und Stoffwechsel, Augustenburger Platz 1
D–13353 Berlin (Germany), Tel. +49 30 450 55 30 32
Fax +49 30 450 55 39 42, E-Mail bertram.wiedenmann@charite.de

Table 1. Incidence and prevalence of functioning islet cell tumors

Functioning islet cell tumor	Sporadic tumors		Tumors in Men-1 % of patients	Ref.
	incidence/ million/year	prevalence/ million/year		
Gastrinoma	0.5–3	4	20–61	5
Insulinoma	4		12–21	7
Glucagonoma, VIPoma, Somatostatinoma			3, 1, 1	8

functionally inert hormones. Furthermore, nonmetastatic, biogenic amine-secreting tumors of midgut origin are nonfunctioning, due to a first-pass effect of the liver, where all active substrate is hepatically metabolized to its inactive form. With the formation of hepatic metastasis these tumors become functioning neuroendocrine tumors, i.e. presenting with a carcinoid syndrome.

Neuroendocrine GEP tumors are further classified according to the location of the primary. They are of foregut, midgut or hindgut origin. Most midgut tumors are primarily nonfunctioning tumors. The prevalence of the carcinoid syndrome in neuroendocrine tumors of the gut incl. appendiceal carcinoids ranges from 1.6% (n = 3,632) to 6.7% (n = 204) [2, 3].

Neuroendocrine tumors may occur as part of the MEN-1 syndrome. Primary hyperparathyroidism, due to hyperplasia of the parathyroid glands, is the hallmark of the syndrome and most often the first manifestation. Single or multiple neuroendocrine, functioning or nonfunctioning tumors of the pancreas are diagnosed in 30–100% of the patients, while 15–100% develop one or more pituitary adenomas in the course of the disease [4, 5].

Epidemiology

Nonfunctioning Neuroendocrine Pancreatic Tumors

The autoptic incidence of mostly small (<1 cm), benign microadenomas is 0.3–16% in unselected autopsies. They account for 15–43% of surgically resected pancreatic neuroendocrine tumors [6]. Nonfunctioning tumors of the pancreas are more common than all the remaining functioning pancreatic endocrine tumor types taken together.

Functioning Neuroendocrine Pancreatic Tumors

The incidence and prevalence of functioning neuroendocrine tumors of the pancreas either as sporadic tumor or as part of the MEN-1 syndrome is given in table 1.

Nonfunctioning and Functioning Tumors of Midgut Origin

The incidence of neuroendocrine tumors of midgut origin is 0.3–0.9/100,000/year [9–11]. Again, the incidence is higher in post mortem examination, indicating that many patients never develop symptoms from these slow growing tumors. On average 7.5 years elapse between the first symptoms and diagnosis [12, 13].

Clinical Presentation

Nonfunctioning Neuroendocrine Pancreatic Tumors

These tumors lack symptoms of hormone excess, thus, the first presentation is related to an expanding tumor mass (table 2). However, with the advent of ever more sensitive imaging techniques asymptomatic lesions are increasingly detected. The rate of malignancy at presentation is up to 60% [10, 14, 18]. With somatostatin receptor scintigraphy (SRS), being routinely used for the diagnosis of hepatic lesions of neuroendocrine origin, the number of patients presenting with distant metastasis may prove to be even higher.

Functioning Tumors of the Pancreas

Functioning tumors of the pancreas present with symptoms due to hormonal excess. Symptoms are similar in sporadic tumors and tumors as part of the MEN-1 syndrome.

Gastrinoma

Hypergastrinemia resulting in gastric acid hypersecretion leads to mucosal ulcerations incl. the esophagus, stomach, duodenum and even jejunum. In addition, secretory diarrhea alone (20% of cases) or in combination with upper GI ulcerations is found. In addition, abdominal pain is observed in more than 75% of the patients. While the symptoms are indistinguishable from those of classical peptic ulcer disease, multiple ulcers or ulcers in

Table 2. Presenting symptoms of nonfunctioning neuroendocrine pancreatic tumors

Observation period years	Patients	Patients (%) with					Ref.
		hemor-rhage	palpable tumor	weight loss	abdominal pain	obstructive jaundice	
9	20	20	40	30	35	35	14
19	9	–	–	–	78	22	15
24	14	–	–	50	57	50	16
15	28	4	7	32	68	21	17

atypical locations, persistence and/or recurrence of symptoms despite adequate treatment, and/or secretory diarrhea should suggest autonomous gastrin production. The mean interval from first symptoms to definite diagnosis is still 4–7 years, and up to 4 years in patients with the MEN-1 syndrome [19–23].

Insulinoma

An insulinoma results in fasting hypoglycemia with Whipple's trias as the hallmark of the disease: signs and symptoms of hypoglycemia, blood glucose concentration below 2.2 mmol/l and relief of symptoms after the administration of glucose. Symptoms of sympathico-adrenergic counter-regulation such as tachycardia, palpitations or sweating may be only modest or even absent. Neuroglycopenia may present as a broad spectrum of symptoms, form slightly abnormal behavior to loss of consciousness. However, the individual manifestation of neuroglycopenia tends to be rather constant. Fasting hypoglycemia or low blood glucose concentrations may occur after prolonged exercise. They may be masked by a habit of frequent meals or snacks. Thus, patients should be meticulously questioned for timing of symptoms and relation to meals or exercise [24–26].

VIPoma

The diagnosis of a vasoactive intestinal peptide (VIP) secreting pancreatic tumor is suggested by a secretory, diarrhea of more then 1–3 l/d (in up to 70% of the patients) persistent during fasting, resulting in hypokalemia and achlorhydria (WDHA syndrome). Occasionally flushing (up to 20% of the patients) may occur, due to the vasoactive effects of VIP. Lethargy, muscle weakness or cramps are related to severe hypokalemia. A VIPoma as part of the MEN-1 syndrome is rare [27–32].

Other Endocrine Active Pancreatic Tumors

Glucagonoma, somatostatinoma or an endocrine active pancreatic tumor secreting GHRH or CRF resulting in acromegaly or Cushing's syndrome have been recently reviewed comprehensively [8, 29, 33]. Due to their low incidence they will not be discussed in this article.

Neuroendocrine Tumors of Midgut Origin

Non-functioning tumors of midgut origin manifest themselves with abdominal pain due to intermittent, recurrent small intestinal entrapment. Obstruction may result from extensive mesenteric metastatic disease, associated with marked mesenteric fibrosis. The primary tumor is seldom large enough to cause luminal intestinal obstruction [11, 34]. A second malignancy develops in up to 30% of patients with neuroendocrine tumors of the small intestine [10, 35].

The carcinoid syndrome is due to the autonomous secretion of serotonin and other biologically active substances by the tumor. In midgut tumors, hepatic metastasis must be present to cause the carcinoid syndrome. Manifestations of the carcinoid syndrome are cutaneous flushing, i.e. a reddening of the face, neck and the upper part of the sternum. A malignant flush may lead to loss of consciousness combined with low or high blood pressure. In addition, diarrhea will be present in many patients. Both, flush *and* diarrhea are observed in approximately 80% of patients at first presentation. Asthma occurs in less than 10%. Together with endocardial fibrosis (30–40% of patients) cardiac arrhythmias and right heart insufficiency may develop [2, 3, 11].

Diagnosis and Staging

Surgical resection is the only form of curative therapy available in localized disease. Hence early diagnosis and meticulous preoperative staging is of utmost importance [1].

Table 3. Sensitivity and specificity of Somatostatin Receptor Scintigraphy in nonfunctioning neuroendocrine GEP tumors (41)

Non-functioning GEP tumors (n = 26)	US	CT	SRS
Primary tumor (sensitivity %)	33	43	79
Liver metastasis (sensitivity %/specificity %)	100/100	83/75	89/100
Other soft tissue lesion (sensitivity %/specificity %)	100/100	78/100	89/100

Nonfunctioning Neuroendocrine Tumors of the Pancreas

Differentiation of non-functioning neuroendocrine tumors of the pancreas from other forms of pancreatic neoplasia, especially from ductal adenocarcinoma is important. Endoscopic ultrasound (EUS) has been shown to be highly sensitive (sensitivity 82 and 94%, respectively [36–38]) in localizing these tumors. Hypervascularization, with resulting contrast enhancement on CT, characterizes neuroendocrine hepatic lesions. Definite differentiation is possible by somatostatin receptor scintigraphy (SRS), since pancreatic adenocarcinomas lack somatostatin receptors. A positive SRS scan makes a nonfunctioning neuroendocrine pancreatic tumor likely [39]. However, the absence of tracer uptake does not rule out a neuroendocrine pancreatic tumor, due to the heterogeneous density of somatostatin receptors on some tumors. The sensitivity of somatostatin receptor imaging is similar for functioning and nonfunctioning tumors. Insulinomas may lack somatostatin receptor 2 or 5, which are preferentially recognized by ^{111}In-pentetreotide, and SRS may be false negative in these tumors [40]. For the detection of local (lymph node) or hepatic metastases in neuroendocrine tumors ^{111}In-pentetreotide scintigraphy is the method of choice. Sensitivity and specificity in nonsecreting neuroendocrine GEP tumors are 89 and 100%. A comparison of SRS, CT and ultrasonography is given in table 3. Following SRS the classification of the tumor was modified in 24% and the therapeutic proceeding was changed in 21–25% of the patients [41, 42]. SRS has its drawbacks. Its sensitivity to localize bone metastases or a primary tumor in patients with metastases of an unknown primary is low [41].

Positron emission tomography (PET) using labeled L-DOPA and 5-hydroxytryptophan (5-HTP) was useless in the detection of nonfunctioning neuroendocrine pancreatic tumors [43].

In conclusion, when the diagnosis of a pancreatic tumor is made, SRS (1) is helpful to identify the tumor as a nonfunctioning neuroendocrine lesions, (2) has a high sensitivity in detecting hepatic and soft tissue metastases and (3) may influence therapeutic decisions with respect to somatostatin analog therapy or peptide receptor radionuclide therapy [44]. For monitoring treatment efficiency CT, MRI or US are superior to SRS, due to their higher spatial resolution capabilities (fig. 1) [45].

Functioning Neuroendocrine Tumors of the Pancreas

Gastrinoma

Fasting hypergastrinemia per se is not sufficient to diagnose a gastrin-secreting pancreatic tumor, since hypergastrinemia does occur physiologically in conditions of hypochlorhydria. To avoid drug-induced hypergastrinemia proton pump inhibitors should be stopped at least one week before the determination of the fasting gastrin concentration. Assessment of the intragastric pH helps to document an inappropriate elevated gastrin concentration in the presence of a low intragastric pH such as it occurs in peptic ulcer disease, either idiopathic or due to a gastrinoma. In addition, normal levels of gastrin are reported in up to 8–40% of the patients at the beginning of the disease [46–50, 111, 112]. If there is only modest fasting hypergastrinemia [<1,000 pg/ml (normal value ~ 100 pg/ml)] a secretin test is recommended for confirmation of the diagnosis. An increase of gastrin by 200 pg/ml or more, in the presence of hyperchlorhydria, will detect 87% of gastrinoma patients with moderately elevated fasting gastrin concentration [27, 47]. Once the diagnosis is confirmed, tumor staging is mandatory. Between 38 and 42% of the gastrinomas are localized in the pancreas, 15–49% in the duodenum, 2–20% outside the 'gastrinoma triangle' (the area between the junction of the cystic and common bile duct posteriorly, the junction of the second and third part of the duodenum inferiorly and the junction of the pancreatic neck and body medially). At presentation approximately one third of the tumors cannot be found, one third is localized and the last third has extensive disease with hepatic metastasis [5, 23, 51, 52].

Somatostatin receptor scintigraphy is the single most sensitive and specific diagnostic tool in localizing the primary (sensitivity 58–78%, specificity 86%) as well as hepatic metastasis (sensitivity 92–100%, specificity 90–100%) [5, 53–58]. Endoscopic ultrasonography is particularly helpful in identifying a pancreatic tumor (sensitivity

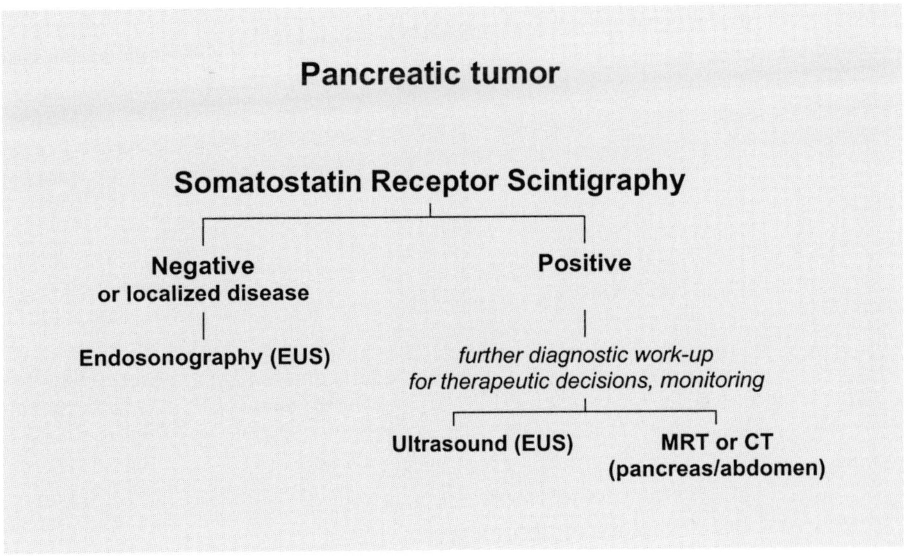

93%, specificity 95%) and localizes about 50% of duodenal tumors [36–38, 59]. The effectivity of both methods is dependent on tumor size. Only 30% of tumors <1 cm are detected by SRS, while EUS may detect lesions as small as 0.3–0.5 cm. Thus, the combination of both may help to increase the localization of small tumors, which can be cured by surgery.

Insulinoma

To confirm the diagnosis of an insulinoma a 48- to 72-hour fast is recommended. A blood glucose concentration <2.2 mmol/l in the presence of an insulin concentration >6 μU/ml confirms the diagnosis in 97% of insulinoma patients [60–64]. To exclude exogenous hyperinsulinemia sulfunylureas should be absent in plasma, and the C-peptide concentration should be >200 pmol/l [65, 66]. In the rare patients with hypoglycemia and low insulin concentration a glucagon test may prove helpful. The glycogen reserve is exhausted after a 72-hour fast in a healthy person, thus, glucagon i.v. will not elicit a glucose increase. In chronic hyperinsulinemia, in contrast, insulin inhibits glycogenolysis, and thus glucagon does increase the glucose concentration (Δ >25 mg%) [60]. When a diagnosis of endogenous hyperinsulinemic hypoglycemia is made, localization of the tumor is required preoperatively. Virtually all insulinomas are localized within the pancreas [7]. Approximately 90% of insulinomas are benign, 6% are malignant tumors, 7.6% occur as part of the MEN-1 syndrome with multiple, small, multicentric pancreatic tumors [67]. Somatostatin receptor scintigraphy often fails to localize the tumor, due to the expression of somatostatin receptor subtypes other than 2 and 5 [61], ultrasonography is recommended as a screening method. In experienced hands, two thirds of insulinomas are correctly identified by transabdominal ultrasound [7]. Endoscopic ultrasound may have the highest sensitivity in detecting small (<1 cm) pancreatic lesions [36]. While computerized tomography is of no help, with newer techniques, such as spiral CT, the sensitivity may rise. Gadolinium-enhanced, fat-suppressed MRI has shown to be highly effective in identifying endocrine pancreatic tumors [68, 69].

Nonfunctioning and Functioning Neuroendocrine Tumors of Midgut Origin

Unfortunately the incidental discovery of small, localized asymptomatic tumors of the gut – which makes primary resection possible – is rare, with the exception of appendiceal tumors. Thirty to forty percent of incidentally discovered neuroendocrine tumors of the small intestine are already multicentric at diagnosis. Generally the primary tumor is too small to be visible on conventional bowel contrast examination. CT with intravenous contrast has a sensitivity of 87% for at least one of three manifestations: primary tumor, liver metastases or mesenteric infiltration. In experienced hands intestinal ultrasonography may be even more sensitive than CT. Due to the high sensitivity of SRS, metastatic disease should be assessed primarily by SRS, while CT, MRI or US should be used to monitor treatment efficacy [10, 11, 45, 71].

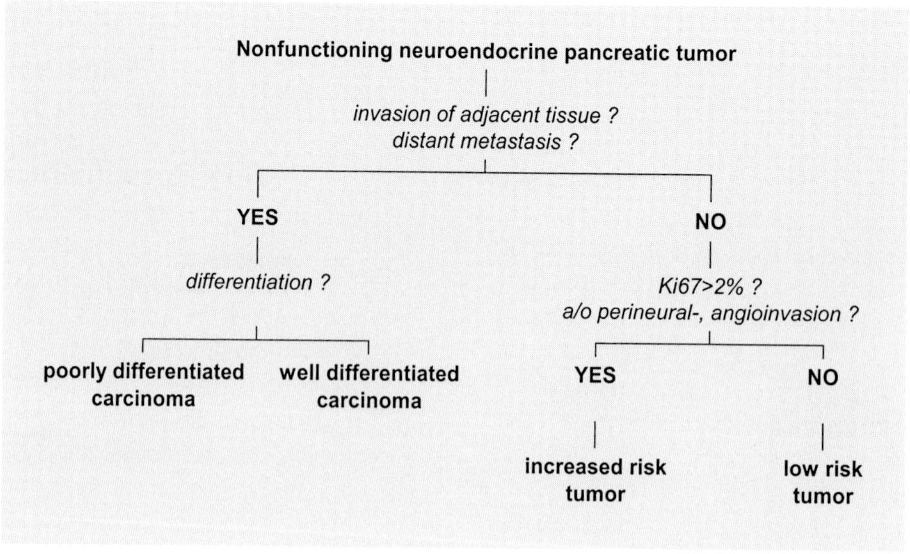

2

Functioning Tumors of Midgut Origin

Endocrine symptoms occur in functioning neuroendocrine tumors of midgut origin when hepatic metastases have developed. Hence, early detection of small, respectable tumors is incidental in most cases. Biochemical diagnosis is made by the determination of serum chromogranin A and urinary 5-hydroxyindolic acetic acid (5-HIAA, sampled for 24 h). To avoid false-positive 5-HIAA results, food containing serotonin, such as pineapples, bananas, or cheese must not be consumed prior to and during the urine sampling [2, 11, 72, 73]. Echocardiography can diagnose endocardial fibrosis in up to 65% of the patients. Endocardial fibrosis may lead to right heart failure. Rarely marked retroperitoneal fibrosis may result in intestinal entrapment or ischemia. For localization and follow-up the same principles pertain as have been summarized for nonfunctioning tumors of midgut origin.

Prognosis

Nonfunctioning Neuroendocrine Pancreatic Tumors

Neuroendocrine tumors of the pancreas are considered slow growing tumors. However, overall 5-year survival is only 44–63% [1]. Their growth characteristics are highly dependent on histological differentiation. Correct staging according to histopathological criteria and clinical extent of the disease are therefore of utmost importance for an individualized therapeutic approach. La Rosa et al. [6] rightly emphasize that the malignancy of clinically relevant, nonfunctioning neuroendocrine pancreatic tumors cannot easily be determined by histological criteria alone, except for those poorly differentiated carcinomas resembling small-cell carcinomas of the lung. Definite criteria of malignancy are gross invasion of adjacent tissue (duodenum, spleen, retroperitoneum) and metastases in regional lymph nodes. Ki67 and vascular and/or perineural invasion were identified as the most sensitive and specific predictors of malignancy. Both were used to classify 27 well-differentiated, nonmetastatic, noninvasive tumors to be of limited risk (demonstrating none of the two variables) or increased risk (demonstrating one or both variables) for malignancy [6] (fig. 2).

In limited risk tumors (LRT) no metastases were demonstrated after a mean postoperative follow-up of 46.5 months and survival was 100%. In patients with increased risk tumors (IRT) metastases occurred after a mean postoperative follow-up of 50.7 months. When the tumor was classified as IRT, well- or low-differentiated carcinoma 10, 34.6 and 100% of the patients died after a mean follow-up of 94, 41.6 and 3.7 months after diagnosis. This confirms the observation that tumor size is of low predictive value in neuroendocrine pancreatic tumors [6, 74].

In summary, non-functioning neuroendocrine pancreatic tumors of low risk of malignancy can be regarded as benign tumors with excellent prognosis. On the other hand, neuroendocrine tumors with increased risk of malignancy can be classified as well differentiated neuroendocrine carcinomas, diagnosed before manifestation of invasive behavior. It follows that treatment strategy for IRT should be as aggressive as those for neuroendocrine carcinomas.

Functioning Neuroendocrine Pancreatic Tumors

Gastrinoma

With the advent of proton pump inhibitors gastric hypersecretion and resulting complications are of low prognostic importance for the patients. Prognosis is worse for those with aggressive tumor growth, characterized by a pancreatic primary, a diameter > 3 cm at presentation, liver metastasis and absence of MEN-1 syndrome. The 10-year survival rate of these patients is 30%. While in those with non-aggressive growth pattern (i.e. 75% of patients) 10-year survival is 96% [5, 75–77]. Patients with lymph node metastases have the same mortality as those who are free of visceral metastases. Patients with MEN-1 had a significantly lower rate of metastasis at the time of initial diagnosis (6%); however, progression of disease is similar to that in sporadic gastrinomas [76].

The level of fasting serum gastrin (FSG) at the time of initial diagnosis correlates often with tumor volume, i.e. the size of the primary, the presence of lymph nodes and liver metastases (as found at surgical exploration), as well as primary site (pancreatic tumors are associated with highest levels of FSG). The 10-year survival rates for patients with mild (0–499 pg/ml), moderate (500–1,000 pg/ml), or severe elevation (>1,000 pg/ml) of fasting serum gastrin concentration are 86, 87, and 73%, respectively [78].

Insulinoma

Five to ten percent of insulinomas are malignant [67]. A high serum concentration of human chorion gonadotropin (hCG) or its subunits may correlate with malignancy. Clinically, benign and malignant tumors are not distinguishable. However, malignant tumors are usually large (~6 cm) pancreatic tumors, and 5-year survival after curative resection is given with 63% or a median interval of 2.8 years [67, 79, 80].

Nonfunctioning and Functioning Neuroendocrine Tumors of the Small Intestine

In extra-pancreatic neuroendocrine tumors restricted to the small bowel wall, with seemingly curative resection, recurrences with metastases occur after a median time of 16 years. After 25 years only 23% of the patients are free of disease. However, life expectancy is normal in these patients. In contrast, when unresectable abdominal or hepatic metastases are diagnosed, survival is only 30% at 5 years. The location of the primary and tumor size are the most important factors influencing prognosis. For localized tumors of the small intestine the 5-year survival is 65–75%. If localized and nonlocalized stages are considered together, the 5-year survival rate is approximately 55% [11]. In addition survival rates may be influenced by a high rate of associated neoplasms.

The presence of the carcinoid syndrome confers a poor prognosis. The prevalence of the carcinoid syndrome is 1.6 and 6.7% in 2 large series [2, 3]. The 5-year survival in patients with carcinoid syndrome is 21% [81]. The median survival is 38 months from the first facial flush and 23 months from the first detection of elevated concentration of 5-HIAA [81]. The prevalence of carcinoid heart disease is 30–65%. With the advent of effective antisecretory treatment, endocardial fibrosis is the life-limiting factor in half of these cases [2, 9, 13]. In patients with local disease, 10-year-survival is in excess of 60%, but drops to a 5-year-survival of 40–50% when metastases have developed [10, 83].

Therapy

Surgery

Surgical resection with curative intent is possible only in patients with localized nonfunctioning neuroendocrine pancreatic tumor at diagnosis. Survival is significantly higher in those with localized disease compared to patients with distant metastases, and further survival advantage is achieved by successful removal of the primary tumor [18]. A recent review cites actuarial 5-year survival rates ranging from 44 to 63% with a median survival time of 30 months to 4.8 years [1]. Data from four series are given in table 4. They show that curative surgery for metastatic disease, i.e. resection of anatomically localized and surgically resectable hepatic metastases can be considered for selected patients. However, this approach should only be considered if the procedure can be performed with acceptable morbidity (<20%) and mortality (<5 or even 1%) [85]. Careful patients selection is important. They should have a resectable primary tumor, but liver metastasis unresponsive to nonsurgical therapy, no extrahepatic lesions and no additional operative risk factors. A recent retrospective analysis (1989–1999) of 41 patients with neuroendocrine tumors of various locations and liver metastases reports that 26/41 patients were treated with hepatic resections, 16 of these with a curative intent. Thirteen of these 16 procedures were finished as R0, 3 as R1 resections. The median survival time after R0 was 70 months, while it was 47 months for those without hepatic resection [85].

Palliative resection of the primary tumor in nonfunctioning neuroendocrine pancreatic tumors has been per-

Table 4. Curative resection and survival rates in patients in with nonfunctioning neuroendocrine pancreatic tumors: localized versus extended disease

Localized disease				Extended disease			Ref.
n	observation time	survival % patients	median survival	n	survival % patients	median survival	
19	5 years	72	6.8 years	20	44	4.7 years	18
10			42 months	10		32 months	14
4	40 months	100	–	9	63	–	84
10	2 years	78	124 months	7	71	75 months	17

Table 5. Palliative surgery in nonfunctioning neuroendocrine GEP tumors

Patients	Palliative surgery	Survival	Ref.
8	4	4.5 years (mean)	86
73	12	4.5 years (median)	18
13	9	63% (at 40 months)	84
20	7	16 months (median)	14
13	7	3 patients (time?)	16

formed. Results of small series are given in table 5. Palliative resection of the primary tumor had no significant effect on patients survival (n = 54, survival without palliative resection 38%, with palliative resection 41%). However, palliative resection may be indicated when symptoms from extensive primary tumor growth become life threatening or unbearable (e.g. gastrointestinal hemorrhage, pain, or gastric outlet obstruction in patients with duodenal invasion). This is different from the situation in patients with functioning pancreatic tumors, in whom cytoreductive surgery may relieve the symptoms of hormonal excess.

In a retrospective analysis of 24 patients with neuroendocrine tumors of the gut (functioning and nonfunctioning tumors), 82% (9/11) patients with curative resection were alive at a median time of 34 months, while in 62% (8/13) patients with palliative resection median survival time was 10 months [87]. In 13 patients with neuroendocrine tumors of pancreatic and midgut origin survival was 91 and 66% at 3 and 6 years, respectively. Disease-free survival was 69% at 3 years. The French multicenter study on liver resection in 131 patients with neuroendocrine tumors reports an overall mean survival of 66 (3–132) months and a disease-free survival after liver resection of 41 (31–120) months, respectively [85]. In the study by Pascher et al. [88] tumor debulking was performed in 10/26 patients. The median survival time after debulking procedure was 50 months. No difference in the survival time of metastatic neuroendocrine pancreatic and midgut tumors was evident [88]. Since patients with unresected liver metastasis are reported to have a 5-year survival rate of only 13–43% [89], hepatic metastasis resection may improve the outcome of carefully selected patients with liver metastases. Unfortunately only a minority of patients (5–8%) are candidates for curative or even palliative surgery because of the diffuse spread of metastases [90]. For effective palliation 90% of the involved liver tissue should be removed [87].

Liver Transplantation

Liver transplantation has been suggested for patients with metastases from endocrine tumors that are confined to the liver. Of 27 transplanted patients, 15 died within a mean of 4.3 months (10 of complications of the surgical procedure, 5 of recurrent disease). The median survival time of the remaining patients was 25 months. It is noteworthy that, although 16 of these 27 patients had been considered free of extrahepatic disease, 8 actually were found intraoperatively to have extrahepatic spread. In a recent meta-analysis [91] 30 cases of liver transplantation for neuroendocrine tumors of different histological types were evaluated. The median follow-up of these patients was 9 (0.3–42) months. The actuarial survival was 52% after 1 year, with 6 patients alive and at risk at 2 years and 3 patients alive and at risk at 3 years. 12 patients died within the first year, 6 of complications of the transplantation procedure and the other 6 of tumor recurrence (possibly in part because of the obligatory immunosuppressive treatment). Thus, liver transplantation for patients with neuroendocrine tumors is presently fraught with both, high perioperative mortality and an elevated rate of recurrent disease (table 6).

Table 6. Results of liver transplantation in neuroendocrine tumors of the gut

Patients	Deaths caused by therapy	Deaths after recurrence		Surviving patients		Ref.
		n	median survival months	n	median survival months	
5	1	–		4	4, 23, 26, 37	92
9	5	1	7	3	15, 24, 58	93
4	1	3	5, 7, 33	–		94
5	1	1	8*	2	23, 41	95
4	2	–		2	20, 38	96
30	6	7	9	117	?	91

* One additional patient died of previously unsuspected cholangiocarcinoma 9 months after transplantation.

Neuroendocrine Tumors of the GEP System and MEN-1

MEN-1 is an autosomal dominant disease of high penetrance, with mutation of the MEN-1 gene at chromosome 11q13 and loss of heterozygosity, that is inactivation of the unaffected allele of the MEN-1 gene. There is no genotype-phenotype correlation [97, 98]. In the index patient the syndrome is usually diagnosed in the 4th or 5th decade of life, however, biochemical evidence in an established MEN-1 kindred may be possible already in adolescence. In addition to the three classical lesions of MEN-1 adrenocortical proliferation (hyperplasia, adenoma, and a rare carcinoma) may occur in 36–41% of the patients, mostly in those with insulin-secreting pancreatic tumor [99, 100]. Patients with neuroendocrine pancreatic tumors should be screened for the presence of a MEN-1 syndrome, as any of the classical lesions could be the presenting symptom [101]. A pancreatic tumor is the second most common manifestation, tumor growth is slow, however malignancy ultimately develops in up to 50% of pancreatic tumors. In pathological series nonfunctioning neuroendocrine pancreatic tumors are demonstrated in almost 100% of the patients, while in clinical series the prevalence of pancreatic tumors is 30–40% [102].

Nonfunctioning or functioning pancreatic tumors secrete at least one measurable tumor marker. In young asymptomatic patients the sensitivity of serum markers is 56, 67 and 60% for insulin, pancreatic polypeptide and chromogranin A, respectively [101]. The time lag between measurable tumor markers and symptomatic disease is about 10 years. At this time point about half of the nonfunctioning tumors are malignant [103]. Standardized screening in these patients enables detection of asymptomatic tumor disease at a mean age of 25 (range 16–38) years. On the other hand, in patients diagnosed without screening, 75% had endocrine morbidity related to the pancreatic tumor and significant incidence of malignant transformation [101]. Thus, annual screening with sensitive tumor markers (chromogranin A or pancreatic polypeptide) is highly recommended. A meal stimulation test with determination of PP has been proposed for early diagnosis with an exaggerated increase of PP indicative of a pancreatic tumor [104]. For intensive investigation to start, two independent tumor markers should be elevated. An increase in hCG or its subunit may indicate malignant transformation [105]. For visualization of the tumor burden endoscopic ultrasonography is the most sensitive (70–93%) single method for pancreatic tumors [106, 107]. Surgery should be considered in patients with clearly elevated tumor markers or elevated tumor markers and visualization of a pancreatic tumor.

Gastrinoma is the second most frequently found tumor in patients with MEN-1 syndrome. In contrast to unspecific markers gastrin is rarely elevated in asymptomatic patients, thus elevations indicate a more advanced tumor burden. In addition to pancreatic tumors, small multiple gastrinomas are found in the duodenum in more than half of all cases. These lesions have a high propensity to metastasize to regional lymph nodes. In patients with the Zollinger-Ellison syndrome, concomitant, large, nonfunctioning tumors do occur. Identification of the gastrinoma may therefore be difficult. Biochemical screening should include nonspecific markers. While symptoms due to acid hypersecretion can be effectively treated with proton pump inhibitors, surgery will rarely cure gastrinoma patients with MEN-1 syndrome. However, early intervention with distal pancreatectomy and duodenotomy may significantly reduce the tumor burden and prolong survival [69, 108, 109].

Insulinoma patients may have multiple nonfunctioning neuroendocrine pancreatic tumors in addition to the insulin-secreting lesion. However, most often only one single tumor is responsible for insulin secretion. Thus, localization of the insulinoma is desirable. Venous sampling or an arterial calcium infusion test may be helpful, however, considerable experience is needed. Alternatively a distal pancreatectomy is recommended, even if only a single tumor has been identified preoperatively. Extrapancreatic insulinomas do not occur. The cure rate is high in patients with insulinomas and malignant transformation of these tumors is rare. Thus, once the syndrome of hypoglycemia due to endogenous hyperinsulinemia is diagnosed, surgery is the therapy of choice.

In addition to screening of the index patient, genetic screening of relatives should be performed. Patients who prove to be negative on genetic testing do not have to undergo further clinical screening. Those with positive genetic test results should be screened annually according to the afore mentioned principles. Malignancy can be expected to occur between one or three decades after the onset of biochemical detectable pancreatic disease. Thus, distal pancreatectomy and enucleation of lesions in the head of the pancreas may help to gain substantial periods without malignant development [101, 103, 109, 110].

References

1 Hochwald NS, Conlon KC, Brennan MF: Nonfunctional pancreatic islet cell tumors; in Doherty GM, Skögseid B (eds): Surgical Endocrinology. Philadelphia, Lippincott, Williams & Wilkins, 2001, pp 361–374.
2 Creutzfeldt W: Carcinoid tumors: Development of our knowledge. World J Surg 1996;20:126–131.
3 Bax NDS, Woods HF, Batchelor A, Jennings M: Clinical manifestations of carcinoid disease. World J Surg 1996;20:142–146.
4 Skögseid B, Rastad J, Akerström G: Pancreatic endocrine tumors in multiple endocrine neoplasia type 1; in Doherty GM, Skögseid B (eds): Surgical Endocrinology. Philadelphia, Lippincott, Williams & Wilkins, 2001, pp 510–524.
5 Jensen RT: Zollinger-Ellison syndrome; in Doherty GM, Skögseid B (eds): Surgical Endocrinology. Philadelphia, Lippincott, Williams & Wilkins, 2001, pp 291–344.
6 La Rosa S, Sessa F, Capella C, Fiva C, Leone BE, Klersy C, Rindi G, Solcia E: Prognostic criteria in nonfunctioning pancreatic endocrine tumours. Virchows Arch 1996;429:323–333.
7 Grant CS: Insulinoma; in Doherty GM, Skögseid B (eds): Surgical Endocrinology. Philadelphia, Lippincott, Williams & Wilkins, 2001, pp 345–360.
8 Doherty GM: Vipoma, glucagonomas, and other rare islet cell tumors; in Doherty GM, Skögseid B (eds): Surgical Endocrinology. Philadelphia, Lippincott, Williams & Wilkins, 2001, pp 375–380.
9 Caplin ME, Buscombe JR, Hilson AJ, Jones AL, Watkinson AF, Borroughs AK: Carcinoid tumour. Lancet 1998;352:799–805.
10 Modlin IM, Sandor A: An analysis of 8,305 cases of carcinoid tumors. Cancer 1997;79:813–829.
11 Moertel CG: An odyssee in the land of small tumors. J Clin Oncol 1987;5:1503–1522.
12 Mignon M: Natural history of neuroendocrine enteropancreatic tumors. Digestion 2000;62 (suppl 1):51–58.
13 Makridis C, Rastad J, Öberg K, Akerström G: Progression of metastases and symptom improvement from laparotomy in midgut carcinoid tumors. World J Surg 1996;20:900–907.
14 Cheslyn-Curtis S, Sitaram V, Williamson RCN: Management of non-functioning neuroendocrine tumours of the pancreas. Br J Surg 1993;80:625–627.
15 White TJ, Edney JA, Thompson JS, Karrer FW, Moor BJ: Is there a prognostic difference between functional and nonfunctional islet cell tumors? Am J Surg 1994;168:627–630.
16 Madura JA, Cummings OW, Wiebke EA, Broadie TA, Goulet RL, Howard TJ: Nonfunctioning islet cell tumors of the pancreas: A difficult diagnosis but one worth the effort. Am Surg 1997;63:573–578.
17 Matthews BD, Heniford BT, Reardon PR, Brunicardi FC, Greene FL: Surgical experience with nonfunctioning neuroendocrine tumors of the pancreas. Am Surg 2000;66:1116–1123.
18 Evans DB, Skibber JM, Lee JE, Cleary KR, Ajani JA, Gagel RF, Sellin RV, Fenoglio CJ, Merrell RC, Kickey RC: Nonfunctioning islet cell carcinoma of the pancreas. Surgery 1993;114:1175–1182.
19 Ellison EH, Wilson SD: The Zollinger-Ellison syndrome: Re-appraisal and evaluation of 260 registered cases. Ann Surg 1964;160:512–530.
20 Mignon M, Ruszniewski P, Haffar S, Rigaud D, Rene E, Bonfilz S: Current approach to the management of tumoral process in patients with gastrinoma. World J Surg 1986;10:703–710.
21 Mignon M, Jais P, Cadiot G, Ben Yedder D, Vatier J: Clinical features and advances in biological diagnostic criteria for Zollinger-Ellison syndrome; in Mignon M, Jensen RT (eds): Endocrine Tumors of the Pancreas. Front Gastrointest Res. Basel, Karger, 1995, vol 23, pp 223–239.
22 Jensen RT: Management of the Zollinger-Ellison syndrome in patients with multiple endocrine neoplasia type-1. J Intern Med 1998;243:477–488.
23 Roy PK, Venzon DJ, Shojamanesh H, Abou-Saif A, Peghini P, Doppman JL, Gibril F, Jensen RT: Zollinger-Ellison syndrome. Clinical presentation in 261 patients. Medicine (Baltimore) 2000;79:379–411.
24 Harrington MG, McGeorge AP, Ballantyne JP, Beastall G: A prospective survey for insulinomas in a neurology department. Lancet 1983;14:1094–1095.
25 Service FJ, Dale AJD, Elveback LR, Jiang NS: Insulinoma. Clinical and diagnostic features of 60 consecutive cases. Mayo Clin Proc 1976;51:417–429.
26 Dizon AM, Kowalyk S, Hoogwerf BJ: Neuroglycopenic and other symptoms in patients with insulinomas. Am J Med 1999;106:307–310.
27 Friesen SR: Update on the diagnosis and treatment of rare neuroendocrine tumors. Surg Clin North Am 1987;67:379–393.
28 Krejs GH: VIPoma syndrome. Am J Med 1987;82(suppl 5B):37–47.
29 Perry RR, Vinik AI: Diagnosis and management of functioning islet cell tumors. J Clin Endocrinol Metab 1995;80:2273–2278.
30 Mekhjian HS, O'Dorisio TM: VIPoma syndrome. Sem Oncol 1987;14:282–291.
31 Grier JF: WDHA (water diarrhea, hypokalemia, achlorhydria) syndrome: clinical features, diagnosis, and treatment. South Med J 1995;88:22–24.

32 Smith SL, Branton SA, Avino AJ, Martin JK, Klingler PJ, Thompson GB, Grant CS, van Heerden JA: Vasoactive intestinal polypeptide secreting islet cell tumors: a 15-year experience and review of the literature. Surgery 1998;124: 1050–1055.
33 Wiedenmann B, Plöckinger U: Neuroendocrine gastroenteropancreatic tumors; in Peckham M, Pinedo H, Veronesi U (eds): Oxford Textbook of Oncology. Oxford, New York, Tokyo, Oxford University Press, 2001.
34 Makridis C, Öberg K, Juhlin C, Rastad J, Johansson H, Lörelius LE, Akerström G: Surgical treatment of midgut carcinoid tumors. World J Surg 1990;14:377–385.
35 Loftus JP, van Heerden JA: Surgical management of gastrointestinal carcinoid tumors. Adv Surg 1995;28:317–336.
36 Rösch T, Lightdale CJ, Botet JF, Boyce GA, Sivak MV, Yasuda K, Heyder N, Palazzo L, Dancygier H, Schusdziarra V, Classen M: Localization of pancreatic endocrine tumors by endoscopic ultrasonography. N Engl J Med 1992;326:1721–1726.
37 Zimmer T, Ziegler K, Bader M, Fett U, Hamm B, Riecken EO, Wiedenmann B: Localization of neuroendocrine tumours of the upper gastrointestinal tract. Gut 1994;35:471–475.
38 Zimmer T, Ziegler K, Liehr RM, Stölzel U, Riecken EO, Wiedenmann B: Endosonography of neuroendocrine tumors of the stomach, duodenum, and pancreas. Ann N Y Acad Sci 1994; 733:425–436.
39 Van Eijck CHJ, Lamberts SWJ, Lemaire LCJM, Jeekel H, Bosman FT, Reubi JC, Bruining HA, Krenning EP: The use of somatostatin receptor scintigraphy in the differential diagnosis of pancreatic duct cancers and islet cell tumors. Ann Surg 1996;224:119–124.
40 Chatal JF, Le Bodic MF, Kraeber-Bodéré F, Rousseau C, Resche I: Nuclear medicine applications for neuroendocrine tumors. World J Surg 2000;24:1285–1289.
41 Chiti A, Fanti S, Savelli G, Romeo A, Bellanova B, Rodari M, van Graafeiland BJ, Monetti N, Bombardieri E: Comparison of somatostatin receptor imaging, computed tomography and ultrasound in the clinical management of neuroendocrine gastro-entero-pancreatic tumours. Eur J Nucl Med 1998;25:1396–1403.
42 Lebtahi R, Cadiot G, Sarda L, Daou D, Faraggi M, Petegnief Y, Mignon M, Le Guludec D: Clinical impact of somatostatin receptor scintigraphy in the management of patients with neuroendocrine gastroenteropancreatic tumors. J Nucl Med 1997;38:853–858.
43 Ahlström H, Eriksson B, Bergström M, Bjurling P, Langström B, Öberg K: Pancreatic neuroendocrine tumors: Diagnosis with PET. Radiology 1995;195:333–337.
44 Kwekkeboom D, Krenning EP, de Jong M: Peptide receptor imaging and therapy. J Nucl Med 2000;41:1704–1713.
45 Ricke J, Klose KJ: Imaging procedures in neuroendocrine tumours. Digestion 2000;62(suppl 1):39–44.
46 Berger AC, Gibril F, Venzon DJ, Doppman JL, Norton JA, Bartlett DL, Libutti SK, Jensen RT, Alexander HR: Prognostic value of initial fasting serum gastrin levels in patients with Zollinger-Ellison syndrome. J Clin Oncol 2001; 19:3051–3057.
47 Wolfe MM, Jensen RT: Zollinger-Ellison syndrome. Current concepts in diagnosis and management. N Engl J Med 1987;317:1200–1209.
48 Jais P, Mignon M: Normal serum gastrin concentration in gastrinoma. Lancet 1995;346: 1421–1422.
49 Jansen JBMJ, Klinkenberg-Knol EC, Meuwissen SGM, de Brujine JW, Festen HPM, Snel P, Lückers AEG, Biemond I, Lamers CBHW: Effect of long-term treatment with omeprazole on serum gastrin and serum group A and C pepsinogens in patients with reflux esophagitis. Gastroenterology 1990;99:621–628.
50 Lamberts R, Creutzfeld W, Stockmann F, Jacubaschke U, Maas S, Brunner G: Long-term omeprazole treatment in man: Effects on gastric endocrine cell populations. Digestion 1988; 39:126–135.
51 Prinz RA: Localization of gastrinomas. Int J Pancreatol 1996;19:79–91.
52 Norton JA, Fraker DL, Alexander HR, Venzon DJ, Doppman JL, Serrano J, Goebel SU, Peghini PL, Roy PK, Gibril F, Jensen RT: Surgery to cure the Zollinger-Ellison syndrome. N Engl J Med 1999;341:635–644.
53 Termanini B, Gibril F, Reynolds JC, Doppman JL, Chen CC, Stewart CA, Sutliff VE, Jensen RT: Value of somatostatin receptor scintigraphy: A prospective study in gastrinoma of its effect on clinical management. Gastroenterology 1997;112:335–347.
54 Schillaci O, Corleto VD, Annibale B, Scopinaro F, Delle Fave G: Single photon emission computed tomography procedure improves accuracy of somatostatin receptor scintigraphy in gastro-entero pancreatic tumours. Ital J Gastroenterol Hepatol 1993;31(suppl 2):186–189.
55 Gibril F, Reynolds JC, Doppman JL, Chen CC, Venzon DJ, Termanini B, Weber HC, Stewart CA, Jensen RT: Somatostatin receptor scintigraphy: Its sensitivity compared with that of other imaging methods in detecting primary and metastatic gastrinomas. A prospective Study. Ann Intern Med 1996,125:26–34.
56 Modlin IM, Cornelius E, Lawton GP: Use of an isotopic somatostatin receptor probe to image gut endocrine tumors. Arch Surg 1995;130: 367–374.
57 Lamberts SWJ, Bakker WH, Reubi JC, Krenning EP: Somatostatin-receptor imaging in the localization of endocrine tumors. N Engl J Med 1990;323:1246–129.
58 Modlin IM, Tang LH: Approaches to the diagnosis of gut neuroendocrine tumors: The last word (today). Gastroenterology 1997;112:583–590.
59 Anderson MA, Carpenter S, Thompson NW, Nostrant TT, Elta GH, Scheiman JM: Endoscopic ultrasound is highly accurate and directs management in patients with neuroendocrine tumors of the pancreas. Am J Gastroenterol 2000;95:2271–2277.
60 Service FJ: Hypoglycemic disorders. N Engl J Med 1995;332:1144–1152.
61 Hirshberg B, Livi A, Bartlett DL, Libutti SK, Alexander HR, Doppman JL, Skarulis MC, Gordon P: Forty-eight-hour fast: The diagnostic test for insulinoma. J Clin Endocrinol Metab 2000;85:3222–3226.
62 Service FJ, Natt N: The prolonged fast. J Clin Endocrinol Metab 2000;85:3973–3974.
63 Fajan SS, Floyd JC Jr: Fasting hypoglycemia in adults. N Engl J Med 1976;294:766–772.
64 Fajan SS, Vinik AI: Insulin-producing islet cell tumors. Endocrinol Metab Clin North Am 1989;18:45–74.
65 Perros P, Henderson AK, Carter DC, Toft AD: Are spontaneous hypoglycaemia, raised plasma insulin and c-peptide concentrations, and abnormal pancreatic images enough to diagnose insulinoma? BMJ 1997;314:496–497.
66 Service FJ, O'Brien PC, McMahon MM, Kao PC: C-Peptide during the prolonged fast in insulinomas. J Clin Endocrinol Metab 1993; 76:655–659.
67 Service FJ, McMahon MM, O'Brien PC, Ballard DJ: Functioning insulinoma-incidence, recurrence, and long-term survival of patients: a 60-year study. Mayo Clin Proc 1991;66:711–719.
68 Thoeni RF, Mueller-Lisse UG, Chan R, Do NK, Shyn PB: Detection of small, functional islet cell tumors in the pancreas: Selection of MR imaging sequences for optimal sensitivity. Radiology 2000;214:483–490.
69 Galiber AK, Reading CC, Charboneau JW, Sheedy II PF, James EM, Gorman B, Grant CS, van Heerden JA, Telander RL: Localization of pancreatic insulinoma: Comparison of pre- and intraoperative US with CT and angiography. Radiology 1988;166:405–408.
70 Cockey BM, Fishman EK, Jones B, Siegelmann SS: Computed tomography of abdominal carcinoid tumor. J Comput Assist Tomogr 1985;9: 38–42.
71 Pae UF, Höcker M, Seuss U, Wiedenmann B: New molecular aspects in the diagnosis and therapy of neuroendocrine tumors of the gastroenteropancreatic system. Rec Res Canc Res 1999;153:45–60.
72 Scherübl H, Faiss S, Zimmer T, Riecken EO, Wiedenmann B: Neuroendocrine tumors of the gastroenteropancreatic system: Diagnostic advances. Onkologie 1996;19:119–124.
73 Stridsberg M, Öberg K, Li Q, Engström U, Lundqvist G: Measurements of chromogranin A, Chromogranin B (secretogranin I), chromogranin C (secretogranin II) and pancreastatin in plasma and urine from patients with carcinoid tumours and endocrine pancreatic tumours. J Endocrinol 1995;144:45–59.
74 Schindl M, Kaczirek K, Kaserer K, Niederle B: Is the new classification of neuroendocrine pancreatic tumors of clinical help? World J Surg 2000;24:1312–1318.
75 Weber HC, Venzon DJ, Lin JT, Fishbein VA, Orbuch M, Strader DB, Gibril F, Metz DC, Fraker DL, Norton JA: Determinants of metastatic rate and survival in patients with Zollinger-Ellison syndrome: A prospective long-term study. Gastroenterology 1995;108:1637–1649.

76 Yu F, Venzon DJ, Serrano J, Goebel SU, Doppman JL, Gibril F, Jensen RT: Prospective study of the clinical course, prognostic factors, causes of death, and survival in patients with long-standing Zollinger-Ellison syndrome. J Clin Oncol 1999;17:615–630.
77 Thom AK, Norton JA, Axiotis CA, Jensen RT: Location, incidence, and malignant potential of duodenal gastrinomas. Surgery 1991;110: 1086–1093.
78 Berger AC, Gibril F, Venzon DJ, Doppman JL, Norton JA, Bartlett DL, Libutti SK, Jensen RT, Alexander HR: Prognostic value of initial fasting gastrin levels in patients with Zollinger-Ellison syndrome. J Clin Oncol 2001;19:3051–3057.
79 Kahn RC, Rosen SW, Weintraub BD, Fajans SS, Gorden P: Ectopic production of chorionic gonadotropin and its subunits by islet-cell tumors: A specific marker for malignancy. N Engl J Med 1977;297:565–569.
80 Danforth DN, Gordon P, Brennan MF: Metastatic insulin-secreting carcinoma of the pancreas: Clinical course and the role of surgery. Surgery 1984;96:1027–1037.
81 Öberg K: Chemotherapy and biotherapy in neuroendocrine tumors. Curr Opin Oncol 1993;5:110–120.
82 Ahlman H, Westberg G, Wängberg B, Nilsson O, Tylén U, Scherstén T, Tisell LE: Treatment of liver metastases of carcinoid tumors. World J Surg 1996;20:196–202.
83 Wängberg B, Westberg G, Tylén U, Tisell LE, Jansson S, Nilsson O, Johansson V, Schersten T, Ahlman H: Survival of patients with disseminated midgut carcinoid tumors after aggressive tumor reduction. World J Surg 1996;20: 892–899.
84 Yeo CJ, Wang BH, Anthone GJ, Cameron JL: Surgical experience with pancreatic islet-cell tumors. Arch Surg 1993;128:1143–1148.
85 Jaeck D, Oussoultzoglou E, Bachelllier P, Lemarque P, Weber JC, Nakano H, Wolf P: Hepatic metastases of gastroenteropancreatic neuroendocrine tumors: Safe hepatic surgery. World J Surg 2001;25:689–692.
86 Prinz RA, Badrinath K, Chejfec G, Freeark RJ, Greenlee HB: 'Nonfunctioning' islet cell carcinoma of the pancreas. Am Surg 1983;49:345–349.
87 McEntee GP, Nagorney DM, Kvols LK, Moertel CG, Grant CS: Cytoreductive hepatic surgery for neuroendocrine tumors. Surgery 1990; 108:1091–1096.
88 Pascher A, Steinmüller T, Radke C, Hosten N, Wiedenmann B, Neuhaus P, Bechstein WO: Primary and secondary hepatic manifestation of neuroendocrine tumors. Langenbeck's Arch Surg 2000;385:265–270.
89 Delcore R, Friesen SR: Gastrointestinal neuroendocrine tumors. J Am Coll Surg 1994;178: 188–211.
90 Que FG, Nagorney DM, Batts KP, Linz LJ, Kvols LK: Hepatic resection for metastatic neuroendocrine carcinomas. Am J Surg 195; 169:36–42.
91 Bechstein WO, Neuhaus P: Liver transplantation for hepatic metastases of neuroendocrine tumors. Ann N Y Acad Sci 1994;733:507–514.
92 Ringe B, Lorf T, Köpkens K, Canelo R: Treatment of hepatic metastases from gastroenteropancreatic neuroendocrine tumors: Role of liver transplantation. World J Surg 2001;25: 697–699.
93 Dousset B, Saint-Marc O, Pitre J, Soubrane O, Houssin D, Chapuis Y: Matastatic endocrine tumors: Medical treatment, surgical resection, or liver transplantation. World J Surg 1996;20:908–914.
94 Anthuber M, Jauch KW, Briegel J, Groh J, Schildberg FW: Results of liver transplantation for gastroenteropancreatic tumor metastases. World J Surg 1996;20:73–76.
95 Makowka L, Tzakis AG, Mazzaferro V, Teperman L, Demetris AJ, Iwatsuki S, Starzl TE: Transplantation of the liver for metastatic endocrine tumors of the intestine and pancreas. Surg Gynecol Obstet 1989;168:107–111.
96 Arnold JC, O'Grady JG, Bird RY, Calne RY, Williams R: Liver transplantation for primary and secondary hepatic apudomas. Br J Surg 1989;76:248–249.
97 Chandrasekharappa SC, Guru SC, Manickam P, Olufemi SE, Collins FS, Emmert-Buck MR, Debelenko LV, Zhuang Z, Lubensky IA, Liotta LA, Crabtree JS, Wan Y, Roe BA, Weisemann J, Boguski MS, Agarwal SK, Kester MB, Young SK, Heppner C, Dong G, Spiegel AM, Burns AI, Marx SJ: Positional cloning of the gene for multiple endocrine neoplasia-type 1. Science 1997;276:404–407.
98 The European Consortium on MEN-1: Identification of the multiple endocrine neoplasia type 1 (MEN-1) gene. Hum Mol Genet 1997; 6:1177–1183.
99 Skogseid B, Larsson C, Lindgren PG, Kvanta E, Rastad J, Theodorsson E, Wide L, Wilander E, Öberg K: Clinical and genetic features of adrenocortical lesions in multiple endocrine neoplasia type 1. JCEM 1992;75:76–81.
100 Skogseid B, Rastad J, Gobl A, Larsson C, Backlin K, Juhlin C, Akerström G, Öberg K: Adrenal lesions in multiple endocrine neoplasia type 1. Surgery 1995;118:1077–1082.
101 Skogseid B, Eriksson B, Lundqvist B, Lorelius LE, Rastad J, Wide L, Akerström G, Öberg K: Multiple endocrine neoplasia type 1: A 10-year prospective screening study in four kindreds. JCEM 1991;73:281–287.
102 Dean PG, van Heerden JA, Farley DR, Thompson GB, Grant CS, Harmsen WS, Ilstrup DM: Are patients with multiple endocrine neoplasia type 1 prone to premature death? World J Surg 2000;24:1437–1441.
103 Skogseid B, Öberg K, Riksson B, Juhlin C, Granberg D, Akerström G, Rastad J: Surgery for asymptomatic pancreatic lesion in multiple endocrine neoplasia tpye I. World J Surg 1996;20:872–877.
104 Skogseid B, Öberg K, Benson L, Lindgren PG, Lorelius LE, Lundqvist G, Wide L, Wilander E: A standardized meal stimulation test of the endocrine pancreas for early detection of pancreatic endocrine tumors in multiple endocrine neoplasia type 1 syndrome: five years experience. JCEM 1987;64:1233–1240.
105 Öberg K, Wide L: hCG and hCG subunits as tumour markers in patients with endocrine pancreatic tumors and carcinoids. Acta Endocrinol 1981;98:256–260.
106 Zimmer T, Stölzel U, Bäder M, Koppenhagen K, Hamm B, Buhr H, Riecken EO, Wiedenmann B: Endoscopic ultrasonography and somatostatin receptor scintigraphy in the preoperative localisation of insulinomas and gastrinomas. Gut 1996;39:562–568.
107 Proye C, Malvaux P, Pattou F, Filoche B, Godchaux JM, Maunoury V, Palazzo L, Huglo D, Lefebvre J, Paris JC: Noninvasive imaging of insulinomas and gastrinomas with endoscopic ultrasonography and somatostatin receptor scintigraphy. Surgery 1998;124: 1134–1144.
108 Grana D, Skogseid B, Wilander E, Eriksson B, Martensson H, Cedermark B, Ahrén B, Kristofferson A, Öberg K, Rastad J, Akerström G: Pancreatic tumors in multiple endocrine neoplasia type 1: Clinical presentation and surgical treatment. World J Surg 1992; 16:611–619.
109 Thompson NW: Current concepts in the surgical management of multiple endocrine neoplasia type 1 pancreatic-duodenal disease. Results in the treatment of 40 patients with Zollinger-Ellison syndrome, hypoglycaemia or both. J Int Med 1998;243:495–500.
110 Skogseid B, Öberg K, Akerström G, Eriksson B, Westlin JE, Janson ET, Eklöf H, Elvin A, Huhlin C, Rastad J: Limited tumor involvement found at multiple endocrine neoplasia type I pancreatic exploration: Can it be predicted tumor localization? World J Surg 1998;22:673–678.
111 Ding W-Q, Kuntz S, Böhming M, Wiedenmann B, Miller L: Dominant negative action of an abnormal secretin receptor with deletion of an amino-terminal exon arising from mRNA missplicing in a gastrinoma. Gastroenterology 2002;122:500–511.
112 Zimmer T, Stölzel U, Bäder M, Fett U. Foss H-D, Riecken EO, Rehfeld J, Wiedenmann B: Brief report: A duodenal gastrinoma in a patient with diarrhea and normal serum gastrin. N Engl J Med 1995;333:634–636.

Review Article

Digestive Diseases

Dig Dis 2002;20:61–69

Surveillance Strategies in Patients after Polypectomy

A. Reinacher-Schick W. Schmiegel

Ruhr-Universität Bochum, Medizinische Universitätsklinik, Knappschaftskrankenhaus, Bochum, Deutschland

Key Words

Colorectal cancer · Polyp · Polypectomy · Prevention · Surveillance

Abstract

Colorectal cancer (CRC) is a major cause of cancer death in the Western world. It develops slowly over several years from premalignant lesions (most prominently adenomatous polyps) to invasive cancer. The molecular basis of CRC pathogenesis has been well characterized. The most effective method to prevent CRC is endoscopic polypectomy. However, adenomatous polyps are known to recur at significant rates. The aim of surveillance programs after polypectomy is to further reduce the incidence of CRC in individuals where percancerous lesions have been identified and treated. However, the medical risks and the costs of repeated examinations must be kept as low as possible. Therefore, the identification of patient subgroups with a particular low cancer risk who may be followed-up less frequently seems important. There is recent evidence that other colorectal lesions, namely flat and depressed type adenomas (F&D adenoma) and possibly some hyperplastic polyps and serrated adenomas may also carry a malignant potential which could influence our screening, treatment and surveillance strategies for the colorectum in the future. General surveillance guidelines regarding these entities have not been issued to date. This article will first discuss the biology, natural history, present surveillance recommendations and future issues for sporadic adenomatous polyps. Then, recent literature on F&D type adenomas, hyperplastic polyps and serrated adenomas will be reviewed with respect to their malignant potential and the potential necessity for treatment and surveillance of these lesions.

Introduction

Colorectal cancer (CRC) is the second leading cause of cancer-related deaths for both, men and women, in the Western world with approximately 30,000 patients dying of the disease each year in Germany alone. Although much has been learned about the pathogenesis of CRC and new and effective chemotherapeutic regimens have been introduced recently there is still no cure for advanced or metastatic disease. Therefore, strategies for early detection and prevention of CRC are particularly warranted. It is well established that the most effective method for CRC prevention is endoscopic detection and removal of adenomatous polyps, benign precursor lesions of colorectal carcinomas [36]. However, the rate of recurrence of colorectal adenomas after polypectomy is high and reaches up to 40% after three years [19]. Thus, surveillance by frequent follow-up colonoscopies after polypectomy is necessary. These follow-up exams may not

KARGER

Fax + 41 61 306 12 34
E-Mail karger@karger.ch
www.karger.com

0257–2753/02/0201–0061$18.50/0

Accessible online at:
www.karger.com/journals/ddi

Prof. Dr. W. Schmiegel
Ruhr-Universität Bochum, Medizinische Universitätsklinik
Knappschaftskrankenhaus, In der Schornau 23–25
D–44892 Bochum (Germany), Tel. +49 234 299 3401
Fax +49 234 299 3409, E-Mail Wolff.Schmiegel@ruhr-uni-bochum.de

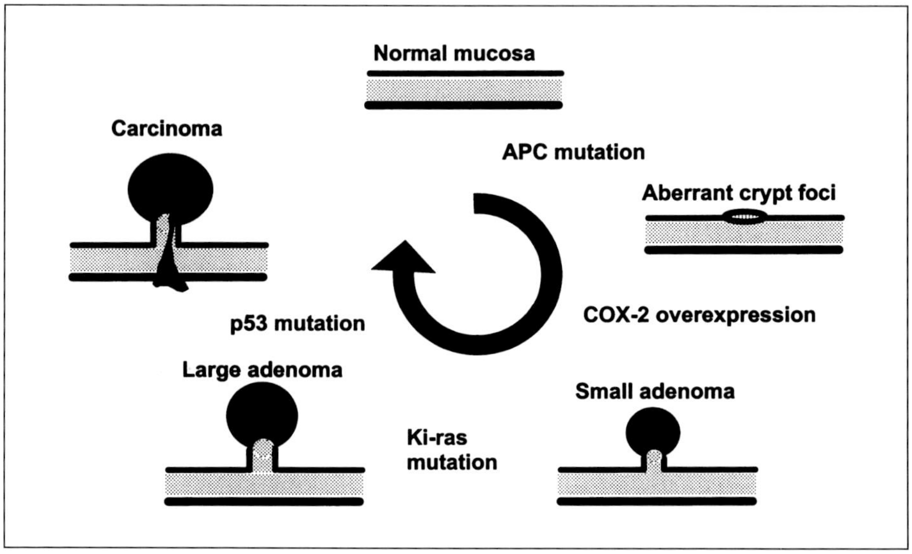

Fig. 1. Schematic image of the morphological steps along the adenoma-carcinoma sequence with its corresponding gene mutations. This pathway of carcinogenesis is also known as the 'suppressor pathway'.

only detect newly formed adenomas but also adenomas missed at initial colonoscopy. Although the benefit of a surveillance program in decreasing the risk for CRC is undebatable such a strategy must also aim at keeping the medical risks and the costs of repeated examinations as low as possible. Therefore, the identification of certain patient subgroups which carry a particular low risk for cancer formation and may be followed-up less frequently seems important.

Recent data suggest that not only adenomatous polyps, but also flat and depressed type (F&D) adenomas [25], serrated adenomas [13] and some non-neoplastic polyps, such as hyperplastic and hamartomatous polyps may carry an increased risk for cancer formation. Thus, individualized surveillance strategies after endoscopic polypectomy for distinct patient groups seem necessary.

Definition of Colorectal Polyps

A polyp is a macroscopically visible protrusion from the surface of the colorectal mucosa and may be classified into neoplastic and non-neoplastic polyps. Neoplastic polyps encompass epithelial tumors such as adenomas, polypoid adenocarcinomas and carcinoid tumors and non-epithelial tumors, such as lipomas and leiomyomas. Non-neoplastic polyps are for example hamartomas (Peutz-Jeghers and juvenile polyps), hyperplastic polyps and inflammatory polyps. To date, only adenomatous polyps have been considered clearly premalignant although other entities may also carry an increased cancer risk.

Sporadic Adenomatous Polyps

Pathogenesis and Genetics

Various molecular, pathological and epidemiological studies have established that most colorectal cancers evolve sequentially from a precancerous lesion, the adenomatous polyp through an accumulation of genetic events [5, 6, 17]. This multistep process of CRC development is known as the adenoma-carcinoma sequence. Recognizable lesions along this sequence are the aberrant crypt foci (ACF), the small adenoma, large adenoma and the invasive carcinoma. Molecularly, the most common tumor inititating event is a biallelic inactivation of the tumor suppressor gene Adenomatous Polyposis Coli (APC), which has therefore been called the 'gate keeper' gene for colon carcinogenesis. Other genes involved include cyclooxygenase-2 (COX-2), Ki-ras and the tumor-suppressor genes Smad4, DCC and p53 (fig. 1). Since loss of function of various tumor suppressor genes is thought to be the prominent mechanism for cancer formation along the adenoma-carcinoma sequence, this pathway of carcinogenesis has also been called the 'suppressor pathway'. Histopathologically most adenomas are tubular, villous or mixed tubulovillous.

Epidemiology and Natural History of Colorectal Adenomas

There is a high prevalence for sporadic adenomatous polyps in the general population with more than 30–40% of $\geq$60 year olds carrying such lesions. In contrast, the life-time risk for developing CRC in the Western hemisphere is only 6% by the age of 85. Studies on the natural history of colorectal polyps suggest that it takes at least 5 to 10 years for an adenomatous polyp to develop into an invasive colorectal cancer. For a lesion ≥1 cm the cancer probability is 3, 8 and 24% after 5, 10 and 20 years. respectively [29]. However, only few adenomas ever become malignant. The yearly rate of conversion from adenoma to carcinoma has been calculated to be 0.25%, certain polyp features significantly increasing that rate. For polyps larger than 1 cm the rate was 3%, for villous adenoma 17% and for adenoma with high-grade dysplasia 37% [5]. The National Polyp Study (NPS) has shown that villous histology and adenoma size are the major independent risk factors for carcinoma development in colorectal polyps while age >60 years was also associated with increased cancer risk [21] (table 1). In this study high-grade dysplasia was used as an intermediate end point and marker for future cancer formation based on data of previous studies by others [14, 17]. The NPS also identified a positive family history for colorectal neoplasia as an independent risk factor for CRC particularly when the adenoma is diagnosed before the age of 60 [35].

Table 1. Predictive factors for malignant transformation (i.e. association with high-grade dysplasia as an established marker for cancer formation) of pre-existing adenoma

Adenoma feature	Risk for cancer development/ Odds ratio for association with high-grade dysplasia	p value
Histology		<0.0001
>75% villous	8.1	
>25% villous	3.4	
tubular		
Size		<0.0001
small (1–5 mm)		
medium (6–10 mm)	3.3	
large (>10 mm)	7.7	
Age		<0.0016
<60 years		
≥60 years	1.8	
Number	increased with number	p = 0.17 dependent on size/histology

Adopted from O'Brien at al., Gastroenterology 1990 [21].

Management of Polyps at Baseline Colonoscopy

These data lead to the recommendation that all colorectal polyps should be biopsied or ectomized in order to characterize their neoplastic potential. Complete colonoscopy is now indicated for adenomas of any size and all polyps should be removed ('clean colon'). Polyps less than 5 mm should be biopsied since histologic grading may be difficult due to coagulation artefacts caused by diathermic polypectomy. Polyps larger than 5 mm should be removed by diathermic polypectomy and recovered individually documenting their localization. However, localizing a polyp by using the length of the endoscope is only feasable in the rectum and sigmoid colon. For more proximal polyps radiologic imaging may be useful. The pathologist should then classify the lesion according to the WHO including the histologic type, grading of dysplasia and information regarding resection margins. The latter may be difficult after diathermy and no consensus has been reached regarding the necessity for a complete resection of an adenoma according to histologic criteria. Furthermore, in case of invasive cancer the malignant polyp should be classified as either low or high risk (see below).

Adenoma Recurrence and Need for Surveillance

Individuals in whom colorectal adenomas have been removed are at risk for adenoma recurrence. The underlying mechanism seems to be an abnormality in mucosal proliferation in adenoma carriers. Some data also suggest that small adenoma may be missed at inital colonoscopy [10].The NPS estimated the risk of adenoma recurrence to be between 32.0 and 41.7% at three years [37]. Similarly, Neugut et al. have calculated the rate of recurrence of colorectal adenoma to be 42% at 3 years [19] which underlines the imminent necessity for follow-up colonoscopy even after complete removal of all colorectal polyps at baseline. However, it has been repeatedly debated whether all adenoma carriers or just certain subgroups of patients should be followed-up periodically. Previous prospective cohort studies had indicated that surveillance endoscopy after polypectomy may only be warranted in patients with certain risk factors, i.e. tubulovillous, villous or large adenomas [3]. The NPS – as the landmark study on surveillance after polypectomy –, in contrast, chose an approach where all colorectal adenomas, independent of size and histology, were followed-up by colonoscopy after initial polypectomy. One aim of the study was to investigate the optimal time-point for the surveillance colonoscopy in a prospective, randomized manner [37]. Patients after polypectomy of adenomatous polyps were assigned to receive follow-up colonoscopy at one and three years (two-examination group) or three years only (one-examination group). Patients who were re-examined twice after screening colonoscopy presented with new adenoma in 41.7% of cases compared to 32% of patients who were

Table 2. Findings at follow-up colonoscopy at both follow-up examinations in the two-examination group vs. one follow-up examination in the one-examination group

	Time point for follow-up examination		p value
	1 and 3 years (n = 338)	3 years only (n = 428)	
Any adenoma detected	41.7%	32.0%	0.006
AAP (adenoma with advanced pathology)*	3.3%	3.3%	0.99

* Any adenoma that was >1 cm or had high-grade dysplasia or invasive cancer. Adopted from Winawer et al., NEJM 1993 [37].

re-evaluated after 3 years only. However, the rate of adenoma with advanced pathology (AAP, i.e. adenoma >1 cm, with high-grade dysplasia or invasive cancer) was equal in both study arms, i.e. approximately 3% [37] (table 2). Only the diagnosis of AAP was considered 'significant pathology' since large or highly dysplastic adenomas were regarded as a marker for future cancer formation as has been previously shown (see above) or invasive cancer itself was already present. Therefore, the authors conclude that 'a follow-up colonoscopy after initial polypectomy at three years is equally as effective in detecting important colonic lesions as follow-up after both one year and three years'. In addition, findings at first surveillance colonoscopy was predictive for future diagnosis of adenoma at subsequent follow-up. If adenomas were detected at first follow-up the patient was more likely to present with AAP at the next examination (after three additional years) than a patient with no adenoma detected at the first follow-up colonoscopy.

The German Society of Digestive and Metabolic Diseases (DGVS) also presently recommends colonoscopy three years after removal of adenomatous polyps irrespective of the size or histologic type of the initial adenoma [26]. If no adenomas are found during the first follow-up examination, colonoscopy may be repeated after another 5 years. In doubt of complete removal of an adenomatous polyp according to endoscopic or histologic criteria, re-examination should be performed shortly.

Issues Presently under Investigation

As stated above, surveillance colonoscopy at three years is presently recommended for all carriers of adenomatous polyps independent of size or histology. However, according to the NPS only approximately 3% of patients are at significant risk to develop invasive cancer in the near future, i.e. those with the diagnosis of AAP at three years after baseline polypectomy. Therefore, some argue that most patients followed-up are overexamined potentially suffering unnecessary colonoscopy associated medical complications such as perforation or bleeding. Furthermore, unnecessary colonoscopies may also cause a substantial financial burden to the health care system. Thus, one of the most prominent issues regarding surveillance strategies after polypectomy at present appears to be the identification of patient subgroups who carry a lower or close to no risk for recurrence of AAP after polypectomy and thus little risk of developing invasing cancer in the future. Thereby, the time period for follow-up colonoscopy after polypectomy may be lengthened from presently three to more years for most adenoma carriers. However, such an approach should only be taken if the adenoma carrier lacks a positive family history for colorectal neoplasia. With a positive family history the interval for follow-up colonoscopy should be kept at three years. That is, of course, excluding hereditary cancer syndromes such as HNPCC where screening should be even more frequent [26].

Factors which influence the risk to recur with AAP after polypectomy to evaluate the individual risk for future cancer development have been investigated. The NPS has already shown in 1993 that although age, the number of adenomas and the size of the largest adenoma at baseline were independent risk factors for adenoma recurrence at follow-up only the number of adenomas at enrollment was an independent risk factor for AAP recurrence (table 3). Recently, another study found that having three or more adenomas at baseline, one of which measuring at least 1 cm significantly increases the risk of important findings at surveillance colonoscopy. At contrast, if patients had two or less adenoma measuring less than 1 cm at baseline the risk of significant findings at follow-up was extremely low [20]. Similarly, results of the Polyp Prevention Study Group also suggest that patients with one or two tubular adenoma represent a particular low-risk group [32]. Although both groups conclude that low-risk patients may have follow-up colonoscopy after more than three years, the identification of more refined markers for recurrence of high-risk adenomas or future invasive carcinoma seems warranted.

Potential Future Molecular Markers Indicating Elevated Cancer Risk

According to the multistep evolution of cancer the biologic and final histologic features of an adenoma are a result of an accumulation of a series of genetic events. Therefore, the molecular profile of an adenoma may provide better insight into its future clinical behaviour than its size or histology. The true profile of a colorectal adenoma carrying a particular high risk for malignant transformation has not been identified so far. Mutations in Ki-ras have been investigated most extensively as potential independent markers for adenoma recurrence or cancer development with differing results. For example, Morris et al. reported that adenomas of patients with diagnosed invasive cancer display a significanly higher rate of Ki-ras mutations than adenomas of patients without colorectal cancer [16, 40]. Other data, in constrast, suggest that Ki-ras mutations are not an independent factor for metachronous adenoma formation [15]. In addition, while some found mutations in Ki-ras to be associated with adenoma features of cancer risk, i.e. large size, villous histology and degree of dysplasia [15] others have only detected partial or no correlation [22]. To date, no single gene mutation is of use to predict recurrence of high-risk adenoma after removal of sporadic adenoma. Clearly, further studies are needed.

Table 3. Multivariate analysis of baseline risk factors for adenomas with advanced pathology* at first follow-up examination

Risk factor at enrollment	No. (%) with advanced features/ No. examined	Multivariate odds ratio (95% CI)	p value
No. of adenomas			
1	1.1	1.0	<0.001
2	2.0	1.3	
3	9.1	2.2	
Size of largest adenoma			
Small	1.3	1.0	0.35
Medium	2.3	1.3	
Large	4.8	2.2	
Age			
<60 years	1.6	1.0	0.13
≥60 years	3.9	2.0	

* Any adenoma that was >1 cm or had high-grade dysplasia or invasive cancer.

Adopted from Winawer et al., NEJM 1993 [37].

Chemoprevention of Colorectal Adenoma and Carcinoma

Chemoprevention after polypectomy to inhibit recurrence of sporadic polyps cannot be recommended at this point although the idea to pharmacologically influence adenoma regrowth after endoscopic intervention seems highly attractive. While several earlier cohort studies have shown a substantial protective effect in particular of non-steroidal antiinflammatory drugs (NSAID) like Aspirin (a reduction in relative cancer risk up to 50%), prospective randomised intervention trials have not been convincing (for review see [12] and table 4). However, promising data from patients with Familiar Adenomatous Polyposis [28] and from animal models of CRC [23] as well as in vitro

Table 4. Examples of trials on chemoprevention of sporadic CRC

Author	Participants	Study design	Substance	End point	Effect, relative risk
Thun [31]	662,424	prosp. cohort	aspirin	CRC death	0.77 (men) 0.73 (women)
Giovannucci [7]	89,446	prosp. cohort	aspirin	CRC incidence	0.56
Stürmer [30]	22,071	randomized, placebo-controlled, followed by cohort	aspirin	CRC incidence	1.15
Giovannucci [7]	25,474	Prosp. cohort	folate	adenoma recurrence	0.71
Baron [4]	913	randomized, placebo-controlled	calcium	adenoma recurrence	0.85
Greenberg [8]	864	randomized, placebo-controlled	vitamins A, C, E	adenoma recurrence	no effect
Alberts [1]	1,429	randomized, placebo-controlled	fiber	adenoma recurrence	no effect

data on new, potent agents indicate that the concept of chemoprevention of CRC should be further pursued. To this aim, future studies should focus on better understanding the molecular biology of adenoma and cancer formation to identify new targets for chemoprevention and on the cellular mechanisms by which certain drugs act chemopreventively in colon epithelial cells. Furthermore, randomized clinical trials should be initiated once promising agents have been identified.

Special Adenoma Subgroups

Flat and Depressed Type Adenomas (F&D Adenomas)

Not all adenomas present as colorectal polyps elevated above the mucosal surface. Some adenomas display a flat or depressed type growth pattern presumably with a distinct biology and prognosis. Although these entitities do not present macroscopically as true polyps we will discuss their common features regarding pathogenesis, malignant potential and clinical management.

Morphology and Molecular Pathogenesis. At colonoscopy, F&D adenomas are recognized by color changes of the mucosa, subtle changes in texture, interruption of the capillary network pattern or highlighting by dye techniques such as indigo carmine. By light microscopy, these lesions are true adenomas displaying intraepithelial neoplasia as a hallmark. Genetically, F&D adenoma carry a smaller rate of Ki-ras mutations than their polypoid counterparts [9]. Interestingly, depressed-type early colorectal cancers as the potential malignant counterpart of F&D adenoma rarely show mutations in the tumor suppressor APC, the major gate keeper gene of classic colorectal carcinogenesis [38]. This may suggest a distinct pathway to colon cancer evolving from F&D type adenoma to flat or depressed carcinoma. In contrast, the rate of p53 alterations, a gene thought to be mutated late in carcinogenesis, is reported to be very similar in polypoid and flat and depressed early cancers as shown by various studies (reviewed in [33]).

Epidemiology and Natural History. The incidence of F&D type adenomas in the Western hemisphere is controversial. Some consider them not a seperate entity but simply very small adenomatous polyps. Their higher incidence in the Far East, i.e. Japan, is by some thought to be simply due to different pathological criteria and nomenclature used among pathologists. However, a recent American study consulting Japanese experts found a significant incidence (22%) of F&D adenomas in a Western population [25]. Two recent European studies had similar results [24, 27]. Regarding their malignant potential, F&D adenomas may contain invasive cancer more often than polypoid adenomas and the average size of advanced F&D adenomas is significantly smaller than that of their polypoid counterpart [25]. It is not yet clear whether non-polypoid (flat) early colorectal cancer indeed develops from F&D type adenomas or, in contrast, de novo. However, the high malignancy rate of F&D adenomas does suggest that flat carcinomas indeed arise from F&D type adenomas [18, 34].

General Clinical Management. To detect F&D type adenomas magnifying colonoscopy using special staining techniques should be used. Presently, it is recommended that even small F&D lesions should be resected because they are more likely to be adenomatous than polypoid lesions. Also, cancer occurs more often in flat adenomas than in polypoid growths as stated above. Depressed adenomas should be treated with an endoscopic mucosa resection if technically possible or by surgical resection. In conclusion, there is still not enough evidence based on controlled clinical trials to issue definite recommendations on the management of F&D type adenomas and more studies are clearly needed. In particular, it is still debateable whether given the malignant potential of even small F&D lesions the general guidelines on the management of small colorectal lesions in general should be changed. So far, at least using special dye methods and/or magnifying colonoscopy for detecing R&D adenoma more easily should be incorporated into general endoscopic practice.

Serrated Adenoma

Serrated adenomas are characterized by a saw-tooth configuration reminiscent of a hyperplastic polyp on low-power microscopy. The epithelium along the upper portion of the crypts is dysplastic. These lesions may also contain tubular or villous components. On a molecular level serrated adenoma show low levels of microsatellite instability (MSI-L) and altered mucin expression. It has been proposed that serrated adenomas are closely linked to hyperplastic polyps and may in fact develop from hyperplastic polyps along an alternative route of carcinogenesis called the 'serrated pathway' which is still being investigated (see below). The biology and management of serrated adenomas will be discussed along with hyperplastic polyps below.

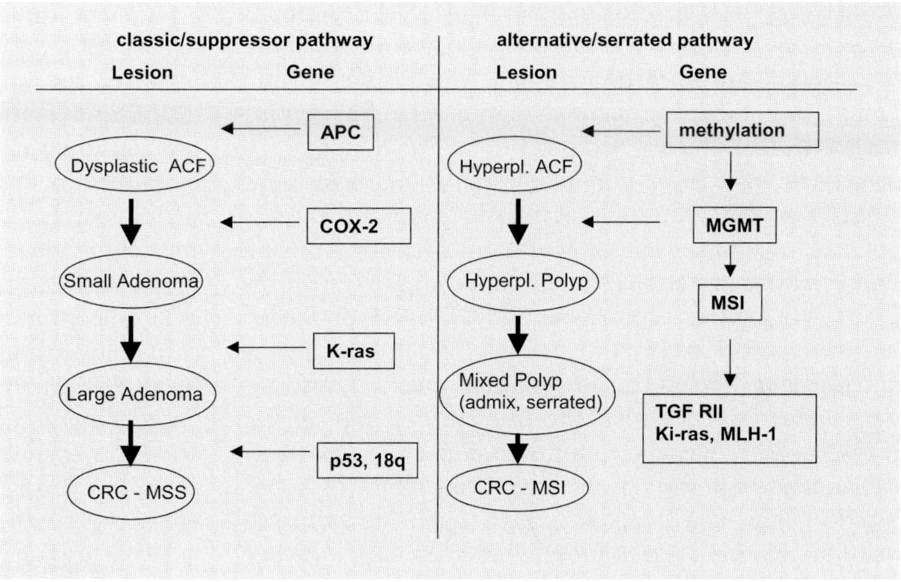

Fig. 2. Proposed separate routes to colon carcinogenesis. Histomorphological entities and proposed mutational spectrum of the classic adenoma-carcinoma (classic/suppressor) pathway and the alternative (serrated/mutator) pathway of carcinogenesis.

Malignant Polyps

If at screening colonoscopy a malignant polyp which has reached the submucosa (pT1 tumor) is detected a thorough histological staging and grading is required to guide further management. The malignant polyp is thereby categorized into a low-risk or high-rik group according to the following criteria: histologic grade 1 or 2 and no invasion of lymph vessels is considered low-risk and may be surveilled endoscopically (after complete polypectomy) at 6, 24 and 60 months. A high-risk T1 tumor as defined by G3 or G4 histological grading or invasion of lymph vessels calls for surgical resection and endoscopic follow-up at 24 and 60 months.

Non-Neoplastic Polyps

Hamartomas

Hamartomas can present as Peutz-Jeghers or juvenile polyps. Intraepithelial neoplasia may occur in these lesions. Sporadic juvenile polyps are composed of large amounts of stroma surrounding dilated mucin containing glands. Intraepithelial neoplasia in these lesions may result from the deregulation of the APC/β-catenin pathway comparable to true adenomas. At present, only carriers of the hereditary hamartomatous polyposis syndromes, i.e. the Peutz-Jeghers Syndrome and the Familial Juvenile Polyposis Syndrome are considered at increased risk to develop CRC. However, these syndromes are extremely rare (less than 0.1% of all CRC are associated with a hamartomatous polyposis syndrome). Therefore, general guidelines for screening and surveillance of these entities can not be issued to date. It is recommended that carriers and patients are treated and counseled at centers specialized in hereditary colon cancer syndromes.

Hyperplastic Polyps and Serrated Adenomas

Carriers of hyperplastic polyps have not been considered at increased risk to develop CRC in the past and surveillance of hyperplastic polyps after removal has not been recommended. However, the prognostic significance of a hyperplastic polyp detected at baseline endoscopy has long been discussed controversially [39]. While some considered left-sided hyperplastic polyps a predictor for proximal adenomas and thus carriers of true premalignant lesions [2], others have not supported this view. In particular, the NPS found no association of synchronous adenomas with left-sided hyperplastic polyps. However, some epidemiological correlations found in adenomas and carcinomas have been described for hyperplastic polyps as well. Furthermore, recent reports suggest that distinct subgroups of hyperplastic polyps may possibly carry an increased risk for future cancer development.

Morphology and Molecular Pathogenesis. The crypts of hyperplastic polyps are elongated, serrated and lined by a proliferative epithelium at the base. The proliferative zone may show increased mitotis. Hyperplastic polyps have been associated with two types of mixed polyps showing hyperplastic and adenomatous features simultaneously. One is the admix polyp considered a histopathological collision of a hyperplastic polyp and an adenoma, the second is the serrated adenoma, which is mainly adenomatous but displays features reminiscent of hyperplastic polyps (see above). Although hyperplastic polyps are usually thought to be non-neoplastic, some have found clonality in subgroups of hyperplastic polyps indicating a potential neoplastic cause. Mutations identified include mainly Ki-ras mutations but also mutations in transforming growth factor receptor type II (TGF-β RII) and losses of chromosome 1p [11]. Interestingly, hyperplastic polyps and serrated adenoma show similar mucin expression which also indicates that the two entities may indeed represent a histogenetic continuum. Furthermore, identical microsatellite mutations have been found in hyperplastic polyps and admixed polyps again indicating sequential relation [11]. Microsatellite instability in hyperplastic polyps and mixed polyps is thought to occur by methylation of the promoter region and thus silencing of certain mismatch repair genes (i.e. the gene for methylguanine DNA methyltransferase, MGMT). Some authors presently suggest that hyperplastic polyps, admixed polyps and serrated adenoma may represent entities of an alternative pathway of colon carcinogenesis, i.e. the serrated pathway, which is supposed to culminate in the development of cancers with a low level of microsatellite instability (MSI-L) and occasionally high levels of microsatellite instability (MSI-H) [13] (fig. 2). This would suggest that some hyperplastic polyps may indeed be neoplastic but do not follow the classical adenoma-carcinoma sequence characterized by the inactivation of the tumor suppressor APC.

Clinical Presentation and Management. Carriers of hyperplastic polyps clearly at increased risk for developing CRC are those presenting with the hereditary syndrome of hyperplastic polyposis (HPS). The syndrome is thought to be very rare but should be taken into account by clinicians dealing with large bowel disease. Patients with hyperplastic polyposis rarely have symptoms unless cancer has developed which means that the syndrome may be underestimated. It is diagnosed if multiple (>30) or large (>10 mm) hyperplastic polyps are found especially in the proximal colon with a positive familiy history of hyperplastic polyposis. Also, 5 proximal hyperplastic polyps qualify for the diagnosis of HPS. Hyperplastic polyposis seems correlated with colorectal malignancy because of the synchronicity of mixed hyperplastic/neoplastic polyps in this condition and the association of the syndrome with the occurence of colorectal cancer.

In summary, there are no general guidelines for the clinical management of hyperplastic polyps and the hyperplastic polyposis syndrome. Small distal hyperplastic polyps may still be considered innocent lacking malignant potential. However, certain features of hyperplastic polyps may indicate elevated cancer risk and should be recognized by the clinician and the pathologist alike. In addition to the diagnostic criteria for the hyperplastic polyposis syndrome listed above these are: presence of high grade dysplasia in a polyp, synchronous adenoma and a first degree relative with CRC. Since neoplasia may occur in these lesions, biopsy or polypectomy is recommended, especially of larger polyps and regular surveillance may be warranted in the future.

References

1 Alberts D, Martinez M, Roe D, Guillen-Rodriguez J, Marshall J, van Leeuwen J, Reid M, Ritenbaugh C, Vargas P, Bhattacharyya A, Earnest D, Sampliner R: Lack of effect of a high-fiber cereal supplement on the recurrence of colorectal adenomas. Phoenix Colon Cancer Prevention Physicians' Network. N Engl J Med 2000;342:1156–1162.

2 Ansher A, Lewis J, Fleischer D, Cattau E Jr, Collen M, O'Kieffe D, Korman L, Benjamin S: Hyperplastic colonic polyps as a marker for adenomatous colonic polyps. Am J Gastroenterol 1989;84:113–117.

3 Atkin W, Morson B, Cuzick J: Long-term risk of colorectal cancer after excision of rectosigmoid adenomas. N Engl J Med 1992326:658–662.

4 Baron J, Beach M, Mandel J, van Stolk R, Haile R, Sandler R, Rothstein R, Summers R, Snover D, Beck G, Bond J, Greenberg E: Calcium supplements for the prevention of colorectal adenomas. Calcium Polyp Prevention Study Group. N Engl J Med 1999;340:101–107.

5 Eide T: Risk of colorectal cancer in adenoma-bearing individuals within a defined population. Int J Cancer 1986;38:173–176.

6 Fearon E, Vogelstein B: A genetic model for colorectal tumorigenesis. Cell 1990;61:759–767.

7 Giovannucci E, Egan K, Hunter D, Stampfer M, Colditz G, Willett W, Speizer F: Aspirin and the risk of colorectal cancer in women. N Engl J Med 1995;333:609–614.

8 Greenberg E, Baron J, Tosteson T, Freeman D Jr, Beck G, Bond J, Colacchio T, Coller J, Frankl H, Haile R, et al: A clinical trial of antioxidant vitamins to prevent colorectal adenoma. Polyp Prevention Study Group. N Engl J Med 1994;331:141–147.

9 Hasegawa H, Ueda M, Watanabe M, Teramoto T, Mukai M, Kitajima M: K-ras gene mutations in early colorectal cancer... flat elevated vs polyp-forming cancer... Oncogene 1995;10: 1413–1416.

10 Hixson L, Fennerty M, Sampliner R, McGee D, Garewal H: Prospective study of the frequency and size distribution of polyps missed by colonoscopy. J Natl Cancer Inst 1990;82: 1769–1772.

11 Iino H, Jass J, Simms L, Young J, Leggett B, Ajioka Y, Watanabe H: DNA microsatellite instability in hyperplastic polyps, serrated adenomas, and mixed polyps: a mild mutator pathway for colorectal cancer? J Clin Pathol 1999;52:5–9.
12 Janne P, Mayer R: Chemoprevention of colorectal cancer. N Engl J Med 2000;342:1960–1968.
13 Jass J: Hyperplastic polyps of the colorectum – innocent or guilty? Dis Colon Rectum 2001;44: 163–166.
14 Lotfi A, Spencer R, Ilstrup D, Melton L 3rd: Colorectal polyps and the risk of subsequent carcinoma. Mayo Clin Proc 1986;61:337–343.
15 Maltzman T, Knoll K, Martinez M, Byers T, Stevens B, Marshall J, Reid M, Einspahr J, Hart N, Bhattacharyya A, Kramer C, Sampliner R, Alberts D, Ahnen D: Ki-ras proto-oncogene mutations in sporadic colorectal adenomas: relationship to histologic and clinical characteristics. Gastroenterology 2001;121: 302–309.
16 Morris R, Curtis L, Romanowski P, Hardcastle J, Jenkins D, Robinson M, Wyllie A, Bird C: Ki-ras mutations in adenomas: a characteristic of cancer-bearing colorectal mucosa. J Pathol 1996;180:357–363.
17 Muto T, Bussey H, Morson B: The evolution of cancer of the colon and rectum. Cancer 1975; 36:2251–2270.
18 Muto T, Kamiya J, Sawada T, Konishi F, Sugihara K, Kubota Y, Adachi M, Agawa S, Saito Y, Morioka Y, et al: Small 'flat adenoma' of the large bowel with special reference to its clinicopathologic features. Dis Colon Rectum 1985; 28:847–851.
19 Neugut A, Jacobson J, Ahsan H, Santos J, Garbowski G, Forde K, Treat M, Waye J: Incidence and recurrence rates of colorectal adenomas: a prospective study. Gastroenterology 1995;108:402–408.
20 Noshirwani K, van Stolk R, Rybicki L, Beck G: Adenoma size and number are predictive of adenoma recurrence: implications for surveillance colonoscopy. Gastrointest Endosc 2000; 51:433–437.
21 O'Brien M, Winawer S, Zauber A, Gottlieb L, Sternberg S, Diaz B, Dickersin G, Ewing S, Geller S, Kasimian D, et al: The National Polyp Study. Patient and polyp characteristics associated with high-grade dysplasia in colorectal adenomas. Gastroenterology 1990;98:371–379.
22 Ohnishi T, Tomita N, Monden T, Ohue M, Yana I, Takami K, Yamamoto H, Yagyu T, Kikkawa N, Shimano T, Monden M: A detailed analysis of the role of K-ras gene mutation in the progression of colorectal adenoma. Br J Cancer 1997;75:341–347.
23 Oshima M, Dinchuk J, Kargman S, Oshima H, Hancock B, Kwong E, Trzaskos J, Evans J, Taketo M: Suppression of intestinal polyposis in Apc delta716 knockout mice by inhibition of cyclooxygenase 2 (COX-2). Cell 1996;87:803–809.
24 Rembacken B, Fujii T, Cairns A, Dixon M, Yoshida S, Chalmers D, Axon A: Flat and depressed colonic neoplasms: a prospective study of 1000 colonoscopies in the UK. Lancet 2000;355:1211–1214.
25 Saitoh Y, Waxman I, West A, Popnikolov N, Gatalica Z, Watari J, Obara T, Kohgo Y, Pasricha P: Prevalence and distinctive biologic features of flat colorectal adenomas in a North American population. Gastroenterology 2001; 120:1657–1665.
26 Schmiegel W, Adler G, Fruhmorgen P, Folsch U, Graeven U, Layer P, Petrasch S, Porschen R, Pox C, Sauerbruch T, Schmoll H, Zeitz M: [Colorectal carcinoma: prevention and early detection in an asymptomatic population-prevention in patients at risk-endoscopic diagnosis, therapy and after-care of polyps and carcinomas. German Society of Digestive and Metabolic Diseases/Study Group for Gastrointestinal Oncology]. Z Gastroenterol 2000;38:49–75.
27 Smith G, Oien K, O'Dwyer P: Frequency of early colorectal cancer in patients undergoing colonoscopy. Br J Surg 1999;86:1328–1331.
28 Steinbach G, Lynch P, Phillips R, Wallace M, Hawk E, Gordon G, Wakabayashi N, Saunders B, Shen Y, Fujimura T, Su L, Levin B: The effect of celecoxib, a cyclooxygenase-2 inhibitor, in familial adenomatous polyposis. N Engl J Med 2000;342:1946–1952.
29 Stryker S, Wolff B, Culp C, Libbe S, Ilstrup D, MacCarty R: Natural history of untreated colonic polyps. Gastroenterology 1987;93:1009–1013.
30 Sturmer T, Glynn R, Lee I, Manson J, Buring J, Hennekens C: Aspirin use and colorectal cancer: post-trial follow-up data from the Physicians' Health Study. Ann Intern Med 1998; 128:713–720.
31 Thun M, Namboodiri M, Heath C Jr: Aspirin use and reduced risk of fatal colon cancer. N Engl J Med 1991;325:1593–1596.
32 van Stolk R, Beck G, Baron J, Haile R, Summers R: Adenoma characteristics at first colonoscopy as predictors of adenoma recurrence and characteristics at follow-up. The Polyp Prevention Study Group. Gastroenterology 1998; 115:13–18.
33 Watanabe T, Muto T: Colorectal carcinogenesis based on molecular biology of early colorectal cancer, with special reference to nonpolypoid (superficial) lesions. World J Surg 2000; 24:1091–1097.
34 Watanabe T, Sawada T, Kubota Y, Adachi M, Saito Y, Masaki T, Muto T: Malignant potential in flat elevations. Dis Colon Rectum 1993; 36:548–553.
35 Winawer S, Zauber A, Gerdes H, O'Brien M, Gottlieb L, Sternberg S, Bond J, Waye J, Schapiro M, Panish J, et al: Risk of colorectal cancer in the families of patients with adenomatous polyps. National Polyp Study Workgroup. N Engl J Med 1996;334:82–87.
36 Winawer S, Zauber A, Ho M, O'Brien M, Gottlieb L, Sternberg S, Waye J, Schapiro M, Bond J, Panish J, et al: Prevention of colorectal cancer by colonoscopic polypectomy. The National Polyp Study Workgroup. N Engl J Med 1993; 329:1977–1981.
37 Winawer S, Zauber A, O'Brien M, Ho M, Gottlieb L, Sternberg S, Waye J, Bond J, Schapiro M, Stewart E, et al: Randomized comparison of surveillance intervals after colonoscopic removal of newly diagnosed adenomatous polyps. The National Polyp Study Workgroup. N Engl J Med 1993;328:901–906.
38 Yagi O, Akiyama Y, Ohkura Y, Ban S, Endo M, Saitoh K, Yuasa Y: Analyses of the APC and TGF-beta type II receptor genes, and microsatellite instability in mucosal colorectal carcinomas. Jpn J Cancer Res 1997;88:718–724.
39 Zauber A, Winawer S: Initial management and follow-up surveillance of patients with colorectal adenomas. Gastroenterol Clin North Am 1997;26:85–101.
40 Zauber N, Sabbath-Solitaire M, Bishop D: Ki-ras mutations in adenomas from cancer-bearing and cancer-free bowel. J Pathol 1998;184: 340.

Review Article

Digestive Diseases

Dig Dis 2002;20:70–72

Chemoprevention in Colorectal Neoplasias: What Is Practical and Feasible?

Luigi Ricciardiello Enrico Roda Franco Bazzoli

Dipartimento di Medicina Interna e Gastroenterologia, Università di Bologna, Italy

Key Words

Colorectal cancer · Adenomatous polyps · Chemoprevention · Celecoxib · Rofecoxib

Abstract

Chemoprevention strategies for colorectal cancer have gained increasing attention. Despite contradictory data regarding the use of micronutrients and antioxidant vitamins as chemopreventive tools, the identification of cyclooxygenase 2 (COX-2) upregulation in colorectal adenomas has led to the development of new drugs, named COX-2 inhibitors, that directly target the molecular mechanism of carcinogenesis. Celecoxib, one of the two COX-2 inhibitors available on the market, has been approved for chemoprevention of familial adenomatous polyposis. In the future, we might expect these drugs to be used in the prevention of colon cancer in patients at increased risk, such as those with a positive family history.

Colorectal cancer (CRC) is the second leading cause of death for cancer in western countries and for this reason it represents a huge health problem [1, 2]. As suggested by colonoscopy based studies, the removal of adenomatous polyps reduces the development of CRC [3], thus leading to a reduced death risk. However, the feasibility of endoscopic screenings and their application on a large-scale population has been quite disappointing, so far. For this reason, many scientists, all over the world, have focused their attention on chemoprevention of CRC and several chemoprevention strategies have been proposed and gained attention.

Chemoprevention is defined as the employment of drugs or natural compounds to prevent the development of benign or malignant tumors [4]. However, in regards to the use of dietary supplements or micronutrients to prevent colon cancer, contradictory data have been produced. In particular, while some studies pointed out that fiber can protect against colon cancer [5], a recent study from Schatzkin et al. demonstrated that the risk of recurrent adenomas is not influenced by a diet low in fat and rich in fibers, fruits and vegetables [6]. Similarly, conflicting results have been produced as for several micronutrients including antioxidant vitamins [7, 8], calcium [9] while a recent study suggests that folate may be protective against CRC [10].

However, a new approach to colon cancer chemoprevention has been discovered based on the first evidence that people with regular use of aspirin and other nonste-

KARGER

Fax + 41 61 306 12 34
E-Mail karger@karger.ch
www.karger.com

0257–2753/02/0201–0070$18.50/0

Accessible online at:
www.karger.com/journals/ddi

Prof. Franco Bazzoli
Servizio di Gastroenterologia, Policlinico S. Orsola-Malpighi
Padiglione 9, Via Massarenti 9
I–40138 Bologna (Italy)
Tel. +39 051 6364106, Fax +39 051 343926, E-Mail bazzoli@alma.unibo.it

roidal antiinflammatory agents (NSAIDs) have a reduced risk of colorectal cancer. In fact, case-control studies have consistently found an inverse association between the use of aspirin and the occurrence of colorectal cancer [11] and lower mortality from the disease among aspirin users [12, 13]. The use of aspirin is associated with a lower risk of adenomas incidence [14, 15], and sulindac, another antiinflammatory drug, causes the regression of polyps in patients with familial adenomatous polyposis [16].

NSAIDs act blocking the enzymes cyclooxygenase I and II (COX-1 and COX-2). Both enzymes catalyze the synthesis of prostaglandins from arachidonic acid. While COX-1 is considered a housekeeping gene, controlling cell homeostasis, COX-2 is expressed at a very low level and can increase following certain inflammatory stimuli induced by interleukin 1 and TNF-α. Recently, COX-2 has been involved in colon cancer development, in particular of adenomatous polyps. Oshima et al. showed the role of COX-2 in intestinal tumorigenesis in mice obtained by breeding APC mutants and COX-2 knockouts. They demonstrated that a dramatic reduction in the number and size of adenomas was obtained in double knockouts [17]. Thus, pharmaceutical companies have developed drugs that selectively block COX-2. These drugs, named Celecoxib and Rofecoxib, have two advantages: first, they reduce the side effects due to NSAIDs treatment, such as GI bleeding, which is mostly mediated by COX-1; and second they selectively block COX-2 which is involved in cancer development.

A double-blind placebo-controlled trial demonstrated that Celecoxib at the dosage of 400 mg b.i.d. and taken for 6 months significantly reduced the number of adenomatous polyps in 83 patients [18]. After these results, the FDA has recently approved Celecoxib as a chemopreventive agent for FAP patients at the dosage of 400 mg b.i.d. As underlined, this has been approved for patients belonging to FAP families.

Nevertheless, it has been recognized that inherited susceptibility plays an important role in familial clustering of sporadic colorectal cancer. The prevalence of adenomas is reported to be higher in subjects having first-degree relatives with colon cancers than in subjects without such a history. In two previous studies we demonstrated that the prevalence of adenomas is almost twice in patients with a single first degree relative affected or dead by colon cancer, and that polyps recur more frequently over a three-year period in this group of patients [19, 20]. Thus, patients who have a family history of colorectal cancer, but do not belong to FAP or HNPCC families, might benefit from chemopreventive strategies with COX-2 inhibitors.

In conclusion, chemopreventive strategies for colorectal cancer have recently gained a big boost. Despite contradictory data on natural nutrient-based chemoprevention of colon cancer, the use of a correct diet, which includes low calories, low fat and high fruit and vegetable intake, is advisable for cancer prevention and indeed important as a well accepted strategy to prevent several other conditions, including cardiovascular diseases.

Furthermore, the use of COX-2 inhibitors to reduce size and number of adenomas in FAP patients has given promising results: this approach might be also evaluated for people who are at familial risk for the development of colorectal cancer.

References

1 Greenlee RT, Murray T, Bolden S, Wingo PA: Cancer statistics. CA Cancer J Clin 2000;50:7–33, 2000.
2 Greenlee RT, Hill-Harmon MB, Murray T, Thun M: Cancer statistics, 2001. CA Cancer J Clin 2001;51:15–36.
3 Winawer SJ, Zauber AG, Ho MN, O'Brien MJ, Gottlieb LS, Sternberg SS, Waye JD, Schapiro M, Bond JH, Panish JF: Prevention of colorectal cancer by colonoscopic polypectomy. The National Polyp Study Workgroup. N Engl J Med 1993;329:1977–1981.
4 Hakama M: Chemoprevention of cancer. Acta Oncol 1998;37:227–230.
5 MacLennan R, Macrae F, Bain C, Battistutta D, Chapuis P, Gratten H, Lambert J, Newland RC, Ngu M, Russell A: Randomized trial of intake of fat, fiber, and beta carotene to prevent colorectal adenomas. The Australian Polyp Prevention Project. J Natl Cancer Inst 1995; 87:1760–1766.
6 Schatzkin A, Lanza E, Corle D, Lance P, Iber F, Caan B, Shike M, Weissfeld J, Burt R, Cooper MR, Kikendall JW, Cahill J: Lack of effect of a low-fat, high-fiber diet on the recurrence of colorectal adenomas. Polyp Prevention Trial Study Group. N Engl J Med 2000;20;342: 1149–1155.
7 Greenberg ER, Baron JA, Tosteson TD, Freeman DH, Jr, Beck GJ, Bond JH, Colacchio TA, Coller JA, Frankl HD, Haile RW: A clinical trial of antioxidant vitamins to prevent colorectal adenoma. Polyp Prevention Study Group. N Engl J Med 1994;331:141–147.
8 Garland C, Shekelle RB, Barrett-Connor E, Criqui MH, Rossof AH, Paul O: Dietary vitamin D and calcium and risk of colorectal cancer: a 19-year prospective study in men. Lancet 1985;1:307–309.
9 Baron JA, Beach M, Mandel JS, van Stolk RU, Haile RW, Sandler RS, Rothstein R, Summers RW, Snover DC, Beck GJ, Bond JH, Greenberg ER: Calcium supplements for the prevention of colorectal adenomas. Calcium Polyp Prevention Study Group. N Engl J Med 1999; 340:101–107.

10 Fuchs CS, Willett WC, Colditz GA, Hunter DJ, Stampfer MJ, Speizer FE, Giovannucci EL: The influence of folate and multivitamin use on the familial risk of colon cancer in women. Cancer Epidemiol Biomarkers Prev 2002;11:227–234.
11 Kune GA, Kune S, Watson LF: Colorectal cancer risk, chronic illnesses, operations, and medications: case control results from the Melbourne Colorectal Cancer Study. Cancer Res 1988;48:4399–4404.
12 Muscat JE, Stellman SD, Wynder EL: Nonsteroidal antiinflammatory drugs and colorectal cancer. Cancer 1994;74:1847–1854.
13 Thun MJ, Namboodiri MM, Heath CW Jr: Aspirin use and reduced risk of fatal colon cancer. N Engl J Med 1991;325:1593–1596.
14 Suh O, Mettlin C, Petrelli NJ: Aspirin use, cancer, and polyps of the large bowel. Cancer 1993;72:1171–1177.
15 Giovannucci E, Rimm EB, Stampfer MJ, Colditz GA, Ascherio A, Willett WC: Aspirin use and the risk for colorectal cancer and adenoma in male health professionals. Ann Intern Med 1994;121:241–246.
16 Giardiello FM, Hamilton SR, Krush AJ, Piantadosi S, Hylind LM, Celano P, Booker SV, Robinson CR, Offerhaus GJ: Treatment of colonic and rectal adenomas with sulindac in familial adenomatous polyposis. N Engl J Med 1993;328:1313–1316.
17 Oshima M, Dinchuk JE, Kargman SL, Oshima H, Hancock B, Kwong E, Trzaskos JM, Evans JF, Taketo MM: Suppression of intestinal polyposis in Apc delta716 knockout mice by inhibition of cyclooxygenase 2 (COX-2). Cell 1996;87:803–809.
18 Steinbach G, Lynch PM, Phillips RK, Wallace MH, Hawk E, Gordon GB, Wakabayashi N, Saunders B, Shen Y, Fujimura T, Su LK, Levin B: The effect of celecoxib, a cyclooxygenase-2 inhibitor, in familial adenomatous polyposis. N Engl J Med 2000;342:1946–1952.
19 Bazzoli F, Fossi S, Sottili S, Pozzato P, Zagari RM, Morelli MC, Taroni F, Roda E: The risk of adenomatous polyps in asymptomatic first-degree relatives of persons with colon cancer. Gastroenterology 1995;109:783–788.
20 Fossi S, Bazzoli F, Ricciardiello L, Nicolini G, Zagari RM, Pozzato P, Palli D, Roda E: Incidence and recurrence rates of colorectal adenomas in first-degree asymptomatic relatives of patients with colon cancer. Am J Gastroenterol 2001;96:1601–1604.

Review Article

Digestive Diseases

Dig Dis 2002;20:73–80

The Role of Genomic Instabilities in Affecting Treatment Responses of Colorectal Cancer

Luigi Ricciardiello Franco Bazzoli

Dipartimento di Medicina Interna e Gastroenterologia, Università di Bologna, Italy

Key Words

Colorectal cancer · Microsatellite instability · Chromosomal instability · Chemotherapy · Chemosensitivity

Abstract

Colorectal cancer is one of the most common tumors worldwide. The knowledge gained on its biology and molecular changes is helping us to choose the best chemotherapeutic treatment. Two different pathways, i.e. the chromosomal and microsatellite instabilities, give the same result but with totally different biological behaviors. In fact, the response to treatment with 5-FU or platinum compounds is dramatically different in both settings. In the future, the use of these compounds should require molecular testing of the speciment prior to treatment.

Introduction

Colorectal cancers (CRC) are the third most common cancers in men and women worldwide. Of all cancer types, the molecular changes leading to malignant growth are perhaps best known in CRC. Combined with a growing number of animal model systems, it has become the most extensively studied human malignancy. Nevertheless, the prognosis of advanced diseases is still poor; at diagnosis approximately one fourth of all cases are stage C, i.e., regional lymph node metastases are present but no detectable metastatic lesions are found in other organs and one third of those diagnosed are stage B2 disease, in which the adenocarcinoma is invasive through the muscularis propria of the colonic wall without involvement of local lymph nodes. Patients with stage C CRC are generally considered to benefit from adjuvant 5-fluorouracil (5-FU)-based chemotherapy, which is often given in combination with leucovorin or levamisole. Disparate from stage C disease (in which lymph nodes contain tumor), stage B2 survival is not improved by adjuvant chemotherapy.

The progress achieved in molecular biology is now helping us to comprehend the differences in chemotherapy response even in tumors at the same stage. This reflects striking differences in genomic profiles. In this review we will report some of the new findings regarding chemotherapy responses and specific genomic instabilities.

Genomic Instability in Colorectal Cancer

Tumors in the human colon have been postulated to initiate as a polyp and progress along a pathway of genetic events to cancer. The first characteristic of solid tumors,

KARGER

Fax + 41 61 306 12 34
E-Mail karger@karger.ch
www.karger.com

0257–2753/02/0201–0073$18.50/0

Accessible online at:
www.karger.com/journals/ddi

Dr. Luigi Ricciardiello
Dipartimento di Medicina Interna e Gastroenterologia
Università degli Studi di Bologna, Via Massarenti 9
I–40138 Bologna (Italy)
Tel. +39 051 63 63 317, Fax +39 051 343 926, E-Mail ricciard@med.unibo.it

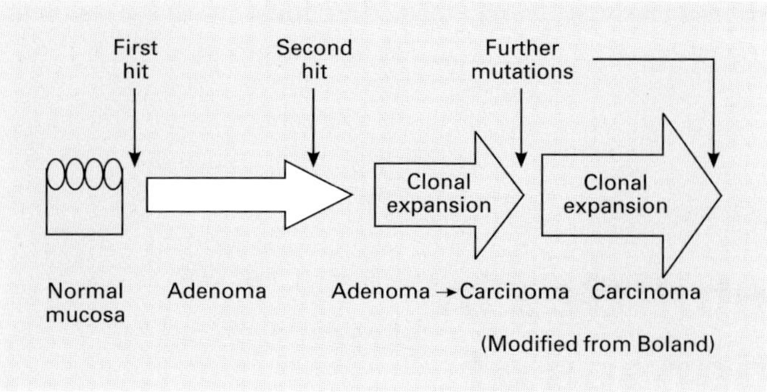

Fig. 1. The clonal expansion theory. Normal epithelial cells develop mutations each day that usually are harmless. However, one mutation can create a growth advantage to the cell. A subsequent second hit can determine a progenie of mutated cells that will develop a tumor.

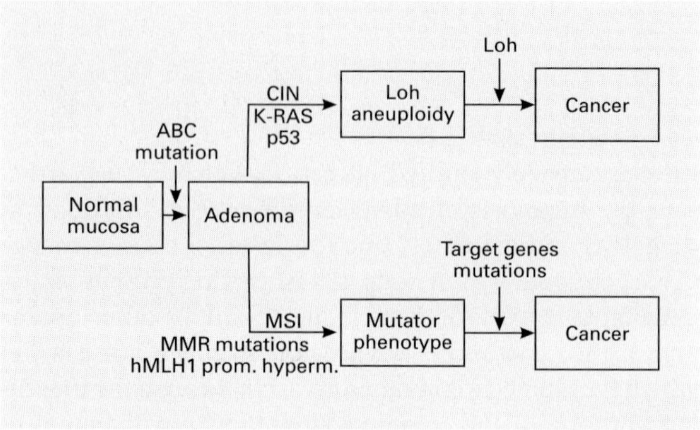

Fig. 2. Genomic instabilities in colon cancer. The key mutation involves the APC tumor suppressor gene. Tumor then progresses through either the chromosomal (CIN) or the microsatellite instability (MSI) pathways. In CIN, K-RAS is often mutated and p53 function is loss, and cells are aneuploid. On the other hand, MSI is characterized by accumulation of mutations in repetitive sequences of genes controlling cell proliferation and apoptosis. In this case, cells are usually diploid.

and colon cancer, is the development of a new phenotype preceded by stages that are often reversible, through irreversible changes that lead to infiltration of the surrounding tissue and frank metastasis. A normal epithelial cell is prone, each day, to mutations resulting from carcinogen exposure or spontaneous mutations. Most of these errors may be irrelevant, or so dramatic to induce the cell undergoing apoptosis. When a particular genetic event creates growth advantage, a newly expanded clone will create a progeny of mutated cells that will induce overgrowth of neighboring cells (fig. 1). This will lead to the tumor formation and this process reflects a situation of genomic instability. The sequence of genetic events leading to colorectal cancer usually begins with the inactivation of the pathway involving the adenomatous polyposis coli tumor suppressor *(APC)* gene and β-catenin. The *APC* gene is obviously involved in familial adenomatous polyposis, but is also involved in the vast majority of all sporadic colorectal cancers [1–4]. In 1990, a stepwise model of colorectal tumorigenesis was developed in which mutations in *APC* were proposed to occur early during the development of polyps, oncogenic *K-ras* mutations arose during the adenomatous stage, and mutations of *TP53* and deletions on chromosome 18q coincided with the transition to malignancy [5]. The *APC* mutation is believed to be the first event in polyp formation, then tumor progresses through two distinct pathways: chromosomal or microsatellite instability pathways (fig. 2).

Chromosomal Instability

The common pathway, observed in ~80–85% of colorectal neoplasms, requires a process whereby chromosomal instability leads to losses of tumor-suppressor genes, characterized by alteration in chromosome numbers through loss or gain of whole chromosomes (named aneuploidy), chromosome alteration, gene amplification and gene mutation. The visible changes in cell morphology and behavior are the direct consequence of the activation of oncogenes, loss of tumor suppressor genes and deregulation of the cell cycle [5]. The *p53*, *K-ras*, and various other genes such as *Src* [6], *c-myc* [7] and genes in the transforming growth factor-pathway [8] are often mutated. In particular aneuploidy is often associated with loss of both parental alleles, termed loss of heterozygosity [9–10]. The mechanism responsible for this form of genomic instability is unknown, which limits our ability to develop preventive strategies for these neoplasms. As previously demonstrated by FISH analysis, loss or gain of chromosomes are 10–100 fold more frequent in colorectal cancers displaying aneuploidy compared to those (nearly diploid) characterized by microsatellite instability [11]. Erroneously, chromosomal instability was thought to be a late event in colon carcinogenesis. If it's true that the rate of gross chromosomal changes increases with cell transformation and evolution through metastasis, in benign lesions such as adenomatous and hyperplastic polyps chromosomal instability can be detected [12]. In a recent report, Thiagalingam et al. [13] proposed a new mechanism leading to aneuploidy that involves chromosome structural alterations rather than gene conversion or mi-

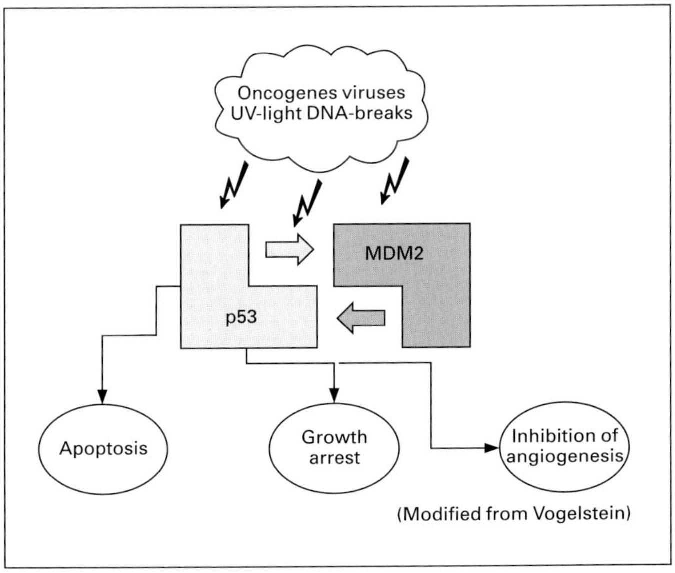

Fig. 3. How p53 guards the genome. p53 is activated by several mechanisms attacking the cell, including UV light and viral proteins. When activated, p53 binds to MDM2 (which promotes p53 degradation), then activating apoptosis, cell cycle arrest and inhibiting angiogenesis.

totic recombination. They suggest that a first hit (such as a mutation in cell cycle checkpoints or alteration of centrosome numbers) would compromise chromosome number in the absence of structural changes explaining the aneuploidy present in benign tumors. The second mechanism would be a defect, unknown yet, resulting in higher rates of structural changes associated with inter-chromosomal recombination.

As mentioned before, some key genes are often mutated in the chromosomal instability pathway, including the p53 gene. This gene, erroneously thought to be an oncogene, was the first tumor-suppressor gene discovered [for review see 14]. When activated, p53 encodes a 53 kd multifunctional protein working as a tumor suppressor in response to DNA damage (fig. 3). This work is achieved by promoting growth arrest, induction of apoptosis and by blocking angiogenesis. When DNA breaks, induced by ionizing radiation, occur, or when the cell is under the stress of ultraviolet light or there is activation of oncogenes, p53 is activated and involves the MDM2 protein in a negative feedback fashion [15]. p53 then binds to MDM2 that subsequently promotes p53 degradation. When p53 is expressed, the protein immediately promotes cell cycle arrest inhibiting CDKs (cyclin dependent kinases) and increasing the level of $p21^{WAF1/CIP1}$[16, 17]. This will arrest the cell in either the G1 or G2 phases, preventing to continue through the S phase or mitosis, respectively. Furthermore, p53 activates the transcription of the BAX gene, which generates apoptosis in cells carrying DNA damages [18]; meanwhile the activation of the gene protects tumor formation by inhibiting the formation of new blood vessels [19]. Chromosomal instability, in particular aneuploidy, has been widely linked to loss or mutation of p53 [5, 20]. Aneuploid colon cancers often display loss of wild-type p53 alleles, p53 mutations or p53 overexpression [21–24].

Microsatellite Instability

The second pathway (MSI) is found in the remaining 15–20% of colorectal neoplasms, and is better understood. The DNA mismatch repair (MMR) system consists of a complex of proteins that recognizes and directs repair of nucleotide base mismatches and slippage mistakes at simple repetitive sequences termed microsatellites [25, 26]. These errors, which can result from mistakes by DNA polymerase, are passed on to progeny cells if the MMR system is defective and may result in insertion or deletion mutations in microsatellites or mutations in key growth-regulatory genes [27–31]. In addition, the MMR system participates in DNA repair during transcription [32], meiosis [33], and homologous recombination events [34]. In humans, MMR activity requires the proper functioning of hMSH2 [35, 36], hMLH1 [37, 38], hMLH3, hPMS1, and hPMS2 [39] proteins; some overlapping functions occur between the hMSH6 [40–42] and hMSH3 proteins because either one may heterodimerize with hMSH2 [43, 44] (fig. 4). Germline mutations of hMSH2, hMLH1, hPMS1, hPMS2, and hMSH6 have been linked to hereditary nonpolyposis colon cancer [45, 46, 37–39, 47], and somatic inactivation of these genes have been implicated in approximately 15% of sporadic colorectal cancers based on the presence of microsatellite instability.

In most sporadic MIN tumors, the promoter of *MLH1* is hypermethylated and the protein not expressed [48–51]. The *MSH3* and *MSH6* genes are frequently mutated as a result of MIN and alterations are seen in late stage MIN tumors [52].

The mechanism for tumor progression has been suggested to be a faster progression to cancer because of a rapid accumulation of necessary mutations in the pathway. The best support for this idea is the frequent finding of frameshift mutations in the transforming growth factor

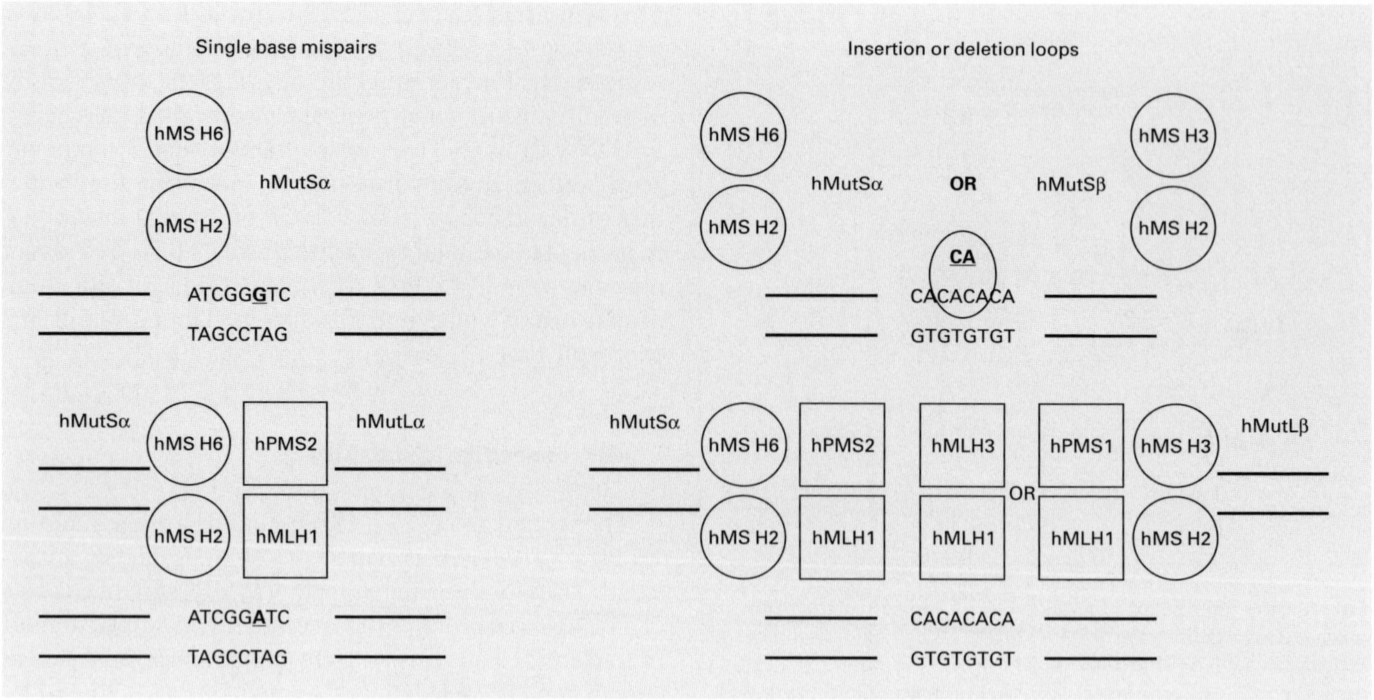

Fig. 4. Human DNA Mismatch repair (MMR) function. If a single base mismatch occur, hMSH2 heterodimerizes with hMSH6 to recognize the single mismatch. This complex, then recruits the hMLH1-hPMS2 complex to repair the mismatch. For insertion or deletion loops, the complex just described can be activated or hMSH2, by binding to hMSH3, can recruit either hMLH1-hMLH3 or hMLH1-hPMS1 complexes.

type 2 receptor in MIN tumors [53, 54], and the repeated clinical finding of clinically advanced cancers within 1 year from a negative colonoscopy [55, 56]. Since all DNA sequences containing short repeats are vulnerable to mutations in MIN tumors, genes with such repeats in their coding sequence are easily mutated and the importance for tumor development is not always as clear as for the TGF-β Receptor II (TGF-β1 RII). Other vulnerable genes known to be mutated in MIN tumorigenesis are IGF-2R [57], *BAX* [58], *TCF-4* [59], *MBD4*, while K-RAS and p53 are usually non-mutated. A striking difference between CIN and MIN tumors is that the latter are diploid, mucinous, usually located in the right colon with a better prognosis due to a lower risk of distal metastases.

Chemotherapeutic Responses of Colon Cancers

Despite enormous progress in understanding the pathophysiology of colon carcinogenesis, advanced forms of cancer remain recalcitrant to treatment. Postoperative adjuvant chemotherapy improves the outcome in stage III colon cancer and is now widely accepted as standard therapy. Many patients with stage II disease are considered at high risk for recurrence and receive adjuvant therapy, although its benefit in such cases is uncertain.

The most widely used drugs in chemotherapy of CRC are 5-FU and its deoxyribonucleoside derivative, FdUrd [60]. 5-FU is a prodrug that is converted intracellularly to various metabolites that bind to the enzyme thymidylate synthase, inhibiting synthesis of thymidine, DNA and RNA. RNA-directed effects are the result of incorporation of 5-fluoroUTP into RNA and subsequent alterations in RNA. DNA-directed effects are attributable to the incorporation of FdUTP into DNA. It is standard clinical practice to administer 5-FU with leucovorin. This treatment leads to stabilization of the ternary complex and hence a more efficient inhibition of thymidylate synthase by 5-FU.

In colon cancer, the need for post-surgical treatment is dictated primarily by the stage of the cancer. For patients with node-positive (stage III) disease, adjuvant therapy with 5-FU and leucovorin or levamisole obtain a 10–15% absolute survival benefit. Long term survival for CRC, despite advances in both surgical and adjuvant therapies, remain in the range of 50–60%. Considerable interest has therefore focused on the identification of novel tumor-based markers that can more accurately predict the course of the disease and helping to determine optimal adjuvant therapy approaches.

5-FU Sensitivity

In the presence of damaged DNA or other stresses, p53, the guardian of the genome, prevents cells from progressing through the cell cycle phases. Its loss can have severe consequences. However, the significance of p53 loss as a prognostic marker for CRC treatment is still controversial. In vitro and animal studies [61, 62] have demonstrated that tumor cells with loss of p53 become resistant to agents like 5-FU. While cells with wild-type p53 are sensitive with 5-FU, which leads to apoptosis, the complete loss of p53 renders cells strikingly resistant. Furthermore, this mechanisms seems to be completely p53 controlled, since the loss of p53 downstream target, p21, does not change the ability of p53 to modulate cellular response to 5-FU [62]. Recently, a report demonstrated that the apoptotic response determined by p53 to 5-FU is mediated by the mitochondrial ferredoxin reductase (FDXR), a gene that contributes to apoptosis with the generation of oxidative stress in mitochondria [63]. The partial targeted disruption of FDXR, with retention of a wild-type p53, lowers sensitivity to 5-FU induced apoptosis.

Furthermore, cells respond to 5-FU with wild-type p53 and overexpression of c-myc. The elevation of c-myc is driven by wild-type p53, with higher transactivation of the first: the authors hypothesized that only patients with tumors showing amplified c-myc and wild-type p53 would benefit from 5-FU based adjuvant therapy [64]. A panel of NCI cell lines treated also with 5-FU revealed that cells with mutant p53 tended to exhibit less growth inhibition compared to the wild-type p53 cell lines [65].

While in vitro data point to the central role of wild-type p53 in governing sensitization of tumor cells to 5-FU, in vivo data are controversial. Ahnen et al [66] reported that patients with stage III CRC with wild-type *K-ras* and p53 would benefit from adjuvant 5-FU plus levamisole chemotherapy. In two studies in which patients received 5-FU, p53 gene mutation has been associated with poor prognosis. The survival rates were found to be significantly worse for those with p53 mutation [67, 68]. Recently, right-sided tumors, with wild-type p53 but showing microsatellite instability have been found associated with survival benefit from 5-FU based fluorouracil [69]. This data indicate that tumors displaying wild-type p53 and eventually loss of MMR function would benefit from 5-FU chemotherapy. In contrast to this data, in vitro studies on the effects of 5-FU and MMR deficiency clearly demonstrate that MMR deficient cells, such as HCT116, are more resistant to the toxic effects of 5-FU and FdUrd. MMR deficient cells also display a less dramatic G2 arrest after 5-FU treatment, which is consistent with the phenomenon of damage tolerance, a hallmark of MMR deficiency. Both studies suggest that 5-FU mediated DNA lesion detection by MMR is part of a major DNA repair mechanism within the cell for maintaining genomic instability. Furthermore hMLH1 responds to 5-FU treatment synergistically to p53.

Finally, a recent report from Watanabe et al. [70] demonstrates that stage III microsatellite-stable cancers with retention of 18q alleles and MSI-H cancers with mutation of TGF-β1 RII have a favorable outcome after adjuvant chemotherapy with 5-FU. Patients with tumors that retained 18q had a five-year disease-free survival rate of 64%, as compared with 44% among those with loss of 18q. For MSI-H tumors with mutation of the type II TGF-β1 receptor, the five-year disease-free survival rate was of 79% compared with 40% among those with no mutation and MSI-H.

Platinum Compounds Chemosensitivity

Platinum-based drugs are among the most active anticancer agents and have been widely used in the treatment of a variety of human tumors. In colorectal cancers, however, cisplatin and carboplatin have been shown to be clinically inactive and have failed to increase time-related survival parameters, either as single agents or in combination with 5-FU [71, 72]. The primary resistance of most colon cancer cells to cisplatin and carboplatin remains poorly understood but is thought to be related to an intrinsically high expression level of different resistance mechanisms including nonspecific inactivation and efflux at the cytoplasmic level, and specific DNA adduct repair mechanisms at the nuclear level. However, compared to 5-FU based treatment, resistance to cisplatin emerges routinely during treatment. The mechanism of action by which cisplatin exerts is function is by determining DNA intrastrand cross-links. Loss of MMR function in HCT116 cells, causes low-level resistance to the cytotoxic effects of cisplatin [73] and renders these cells hypersensitive to its mutagenic effects [74, 75]. This is due by the reduced ability of the cells to sense the presence of adducts in DNA [76, 77].

Using both in vitro and in vivo models, the degree of resistance is great enough that subsequent treatment with cisplatin enriches for these genomically unstable cells [78].

Conflicting data have been reported on the role of p53 and chemoresistance to cisplatin. Some investigators have reported that loss of p53 function renders cells hypersensitive while others have found that it renders them resistant even when MMR is intact [79–81]. Cisplatin exposure induces an increase in p53 and activates G1 checkpoint in the p53+/MMR+ cells. Both p53 and MMR may play a role in preventing the mutagenic bypass replication due to polymerase errors. Although a central role for p53 in mediating activation of the caspase (pro apoptosis) cascade after DNA damage has been extensively reported, and cisplatin evokes a large increase in p53 level in p53+/MMR+ (HCT116 + Chromosome 3) cell lines, any proapoptotic effect of this change is apparently offset in these cells by other antiapoptotic roles played by this protein. In the absence of functional MMR, these cells appear to be more dependent on this protective effect of p53, as the impact of the loss of p53 was substantially larger in MMR deficient than MMR proficient cells. Loss of p53 has relatively little effect in MMR-proficient cells but confers hypersensitivity in MMR deficient cells. Cisplatin exposure induces an increase in p53 and activates G1 checkpoint in the p53+/MMR+ cells. Both p53 and MMR may play a role in preventing the mutagenic bypass replication due to polymerase errors.

On the other hand, the activity of oxaliplatin against colon cancers has been recognized both in vitro and in vivo, as well as in clinical studies. Although differences between oxaliplatin and cisplatin in DNA binding, adduct formation, strand breaks, and apoptosis have been reported, the mechanisms behind the more potent cytotoxic activity of oxaliplatin have not completely understood. Oxaliplatin-induced DNA damage appears to be more potent that of cisplatin in eliciting cytotoxic effects [82]. Resistant to platinum anticancer agents can result from and increased ability of the cells to tolerate platinum-DNA adducts. In vitro and preclinical experiments have hown that MLH1, MSH2 and MSH6 deficient cells, which are resistant to cisplatin, are susceptible to oxaliplatin [83, 84, 78]. The mechanism of action downstream of MMR leading to cisplatin cytotoxicity is not known. Interestingly, the MMR protein hMutSα (which is the result of heterodimerization between hMSH2 and hMSH6) binds to cisplatin adducts but not to oxaliplatin adducts [85].

Conclusion

There is growing evidence that disease-free survival after chemotherapy for colon cancer is determined by specific genetic alterations. For 5-FU based treatments, retention of p53, retention of 18q allele in MSS tumors and mutation of TGFβ1-RII in MSI tumors predict a favorable outcome. Thus, the use of this class of compounds should be determined by testing the tumors for these specific genetic markers. As for platinum compounds, while there is wide evidence that MSI tumors are resistant to cisplatin, there is growing evidence that these type of tumors might benefit of treatment with oxaliplatin. Preclinical studies showing marked synergistic effects with 5-FU encourage clinical oxaliplatin-based combination chemotherapy [86]. The testing for MSI positive tumors should be performed in view of the chemosensitivity of MSI tumors to oxaliplatin before starting treatment.

References

1 Huang J, Papadopoulos N, McKinley AJ, et al: APC mutations in colorectal tumors with mismatch repair deficiency. Proc Natl Acad Sci USA 1996;93:9049–9054.
2 Konishi M, Kikuchi-Yanoshita R, Tanaka K, et al: Molecular nature of colon tumors in hereditary nonpolyposis colon cancer, familial polyposis, and sporadic colon cancer. Gastroenterology 1996;111:307–317.
3 Olschwang S, Hamelin R, Laurent-Puig P, et al: Alternative genetic pathways in colorectal carcinogenesis. Proc Natl Acad Sci USA 1997;94: 12122–12127.
4 Salahshor S, Kressner U, Påhlman L, et al: Colorectal cancer with and without microsatellite instability involves different genes. Genes Chromosome Cancer 1999;26:247–252.
5 Fearon ER, Vogelstein B: A genetic model for colorectal tumorigenesis. Cell 1990;61:759–767.
6 Irby RB, Mao W, Coppola D, et al: Activating SRC mutations in a subset of advanced human colon cancers. Nat Genet 1999;21:187–190.
7 Sarraf P, Mueller E, Smith WM, et al: Loss-of-function mutations in PPAR-gamma. Mol Cell 1999;97:3352–3357.
8 Zhou S, Kinzler KW, Vogelstein B: Going mad with SMADs. N Engl J Med 1999;34:144–145.
9 Vogelstein B, Fearon ER, Kern SE, Hamilton SR, Preisinger AC, Nakamura Y, White R: Allelotype of colorectal carcinomas. Science 1989;244:207–211.
10 Cavenee WK, Dryja TP, Phillips RA, Benedict WF, Godbout R, Gallie BL, Murphree AL, Strong LC, White RL: Expression of recessive alleles by chromosomal mechanisms in retinoblastoma. Nature 1983;305:779–784.
11 Lengauer C, Kindler KW, Vogelstein B: Genetic instability in colorectal cancers. Nature 1997;386:623–627.

12 Staler DL, Chen N, Basik M, Kahlenberg MS, Rodriguez-Bigas MA, Petrelli NJ, Anderson GR: The onset and extent of genomic instability in sporadic colorectal tumor progression. Proc Natl Acad Sci USA 1999;96:15121–15126.
13 Thiagalingham S, Laken S, Willson JKV, Markowitz SD, Kinzler KW, Vogelstein B, Lengauer C: Mechanisms underlying losses of heterozygosity in human colorectal cancers. Proc Natl Acad Sci USA. 2001;98(5):2698–2702.
14 Hollstein M, Hergenhahn M, Yang Q, Bartsch H, Wang ZQ, Hainaut P: New approaches to understanding p53 gene tumor mutation spectra. Mutat Res 1999;431:199–209.
15 Momand J, Wu HH, Dasgupta G: MDM2–master regulator of the p53 tumor suppressor protein. Gene 2000;242:15–29.
16 Agarwal ML, Agarwal A, Taylor WR, Stark GR: p53 controls both the G2/M and the G1 cell cycle checkpoints and mediates reversible growth arrest in human fibroblasts. Proc Natl Acad Sci USA 1995;92:8493–8497.
17 Brown JP, Wei W, Sedivy JM: Bypass of senescence after disruption of p21CIP1/WAF1 gene in normal diploid human fibroblasts. Science 1997;277:831–834.
18 Reed JC: Dysregulation of apoptosis in cancer. J Clin Oncol 1999;17:2941–2953.
19 Hendrix MJ: De-mystifying the mechanism(s) of maspin. Nat Med 2000;6:374–376.
20 Vogelstein B, Fearon ER, Hamilton SR, Kern SE, Preisinger AC, Leppert M, Nakamura Y, White R, Smits AM, Bos JL: Genetic alterations during colorectal-tumor development. N Engl J Med 1988;319:525–532.
21 Bosari S, Viale G, Bossi P, Maggioni M, Coggi G, Murray JJ, Lee AK: Cytoplasmic accumulation of p53 protein: An independent prognostic indicator in colorectal adenocarcinomas. J Natl Cancer Inst 1994;86:681–687.
22 Sun XF, Carstensen JM, Zhang H, Stal O, Wingren S, Hatschek T, Nordenskjold B: Prognostic significance of cytoplasmic p53 oncoprotein in colorectal adenocarcinoma. Lancet 1992;340:1369–1373.
23 Levine AJ, Momand J, Finlay CA: The p53 tumour suppressor gene. Nature 1991;351: 453–456.
24 Goh HS, Yao J, Smith DR: p53 point mutation and survival in colorectal cancer patients. Cancer Res 1995;55:5217–5221.
25 Marra G, Boland CR: DNA repair and colorectal cancer. Gastroenterol Clin North Am 1996; 25(4):755–772;58.
26 Marra G, Boland CR: Hereditary nonpolyposis colorectal cancer: the syndrome, the genes, and historical perspectives. J Natl Cancer Inst. 1995;87(15):1114–1125.
27 Thibodeau SN, Bren G, Schaid D: Microsatellite instability in cancer of the proximal colon. Science 1993;260:816–819.
28 Markowitz S, Wang J, Myeroff L, Parsons R, Sun LZ, Lutterbaugh J, Fan RS, Zborowska E, Kinzler KW, Vogelstein B, Brattain M, Willson JKV: Inactivation of the type II TGF-receptor in colon cancer cells with microsatellite instability. Science 1995;268:1336–1338.
29 Souza RF, Appel R, Yin J, Wang S, Smolinski KN, Abraham JM, Zou TT, Shi YQ, Lei J, Cottrell J, Cymes K, Biden K, Simms L, Leggett B, Lynch PM, Frazier M, Powell SM, Harpaz N, Sugimura H, Young J, Meltzer SJ: Microsatellite instability in the insulin-like growth factor receptor gene in gastrointestinal tumours. Nat Genet 1996;14:255–257.
30 Rampino N, Yamamoto H, Ionov Y, Li Y, Sawai H, Reed JC, Perucho M: Somatic frameshift mutations in the BAX gene in colon cancers of the microsatellite mutator phenotype. Science 1997;275:967–969.
31 Malkhosyan S, Rampino N, Yamamoto H, Perucho M: Frameshift mutator mutations. Nature 1996;382:499–500.
32 Mellon I, Rajpal DK, Koi M, Boland CR, Champe GN: Transcription-coupled repair deficiency and mutations in human mismatch repair genes. Science 1996;272:557–560.
33 Arnheim N, Shibata D: DNA mismatch repair in mammals: role in disease and meiosis. Curr Opin Genet Dev 1997;7:364–370.
34 Selva EM, New L, Crouse GF, Lahue RS: Mismatch correction acts as a barrier to homeologous recombination in Saccharomyces cerevisiae. Genetics 1995;139:1175–1188.
35 Leach FS, Nicolaides NC, Papadopoulos N, Liu B, Jen J, Parsons R, Peltomaki P, Sistonen P, Aaltonen LA, Nystrom-Lahti M, Guan X-Y, Zhang J, Meltzer PS, Yu J-W, Kao F-T, Chen DJ, Cerosaletti KM, Fournier REK, Todd S, Lewis T, Leach RJ, Naylor SL, Weissenbach J, Mecklin J-P, Jarvinen H, Petersen GM, Hamilton SR, Green J, Jass J, Watson P, Lynch HT, Trent JM, de la Chapelle A, Kinzler KW, Volgelstein B: Mutations of a mutS homolog in hereditary nonpolyposis colorectal cancer. Cell 1993;75:1215–1225.
36 Fishel R, Lescoe MK, Rao MRS, Copeland NG, Jenkins NA, Garber J, Kane MR: The human mutator gene homolog MSH2 and its association with hereditary nonpolyposis colon cancer. Cell 1993;75:1027–1038.
37 Papadopoulos N, Nicolaides NC, Wei Y-F, Ruben SM, Carter KC, Rosen CA, Haseltine WA, Fleischmann RD, Fraser CM, Adams MD, Venter JC, Hamilton SR, Petersen GM, Watson P, Lynch HT, Peltomaki P, Mecklin J-P, de la Chapelle A, Kinzler KW, Vogelstein B: Mutation of a mutL homolog in hereditary colon cancer. Science 1994;263:1625–1629.
38 Bronner CE, Baker SM, Morrison PT, Warren G, Smith LG, Lescoe MK, Kane M, Earabino C, Lipford J, Lindblom A, Tannergard P, Bollag RJ, Godwin AR, Ward D, Nordenskjold M, Fishel R, Kolodner R, Liskay RM: Mutation in the DNA mismatch repair homologue hMLH1 is associated with hereditary nonpolyposis colon cancer. Nature 1994;368:258–261.
39 Nicolaides NC, Papadopoulos N, Liu B, Wei Y-F, Carter KC, Ruben SM, Rosen CA, Haseltine WA, Fleischmann RD, Fraser CM, Adams MD, Venter JC, Dunlop MG, Hamilton SR, Peteresen GM, de la Chapelle A, Vogelstein B, Kinzler KW: Mutations of two PMS homologues in hereditary nonpolyposis colon cancer. Nature 1994;371:75–80.
40 Drummond JT, Li G-M, Longley MJ, Modrich P: Isolation of an hMSH2-p160 heterodimer that restores DNA mismatch repair to tumor cells. Science 1995;268:1909–1912.
41 Palombo F, Gallinari P, Iaccarino I, Lettieri TM, D'Arrigo A, Truong O, Hsuan JJ, Jiricny J: GTBP, a 160-kilodalton protein essential for mismatch-binding activity in human cells. Science 1995;268:1912–1914.
42 Papadopoulos N, Nicolaides NC, Liu B, Parsons R, Lengauer C, Palombo F, D'Arrigo A, Markowitz S, Willson JKV, Kinzler KW, Jiricny J, Vogelstein B: Mutations of GTBP in genetically unstable cells. Science 1995;268: 1915–1917.
43 Palombo F, Iaccarino I, Nakajima E, Ikejima M, Shimada T, Jiricny J: hMutS, a heterodimer of hMSH2 and hMSH3, binds to insertion/deletion loops in DNA. Curr Biol 1996;6: 1181–1184.
44 Acharya S, Wilson T, Gradia S, Kane MF, Guerrette S, Marsischky GT, Kolodner R, Fishel R: hMSH2 forms specific mispair-binding complexes with hMSH3 and hMSH6. Proc Natl Acad Sci USA 1996;93:13629–13634.
45 Leach FS, Nicolaides NC, Papadopoulos N, Liu B, Jen J, Parsons R, Peltomaki P, Sistonen P, Aaltonen LA, Nystrom-Lahti M, Guan X-Y, Zhang J, Meltzer PS, Yu J-W, Kao F-T, Chen DJ, Cerosaletti KM, Fournier REK, Todd S, Lewis T, Leach RJ, Naylor SL, Weissenbach J, Mecklin J-P, Jarvinen H, Petersen GM, Hamilton SR, Green J, Jass J, Watson P, Lynch HT, Trent JM, de la Chapelle A, Kinzler KW, Volgelstein B: Mutations of a mutS homolog in hereditary nonpolyposis colorectal cancer. Cell 1993;75:1215–1225.
46 Fishel R, Lescoe MK, Rao MRS, Copeland NG, Jenkins NA, Garber J, Kane MR: The human mutator gene homolog MSH2 and its association with hereditary nonpolyposis colon cancer. Cell 1993;75:1027–1038.
47 Akiyama Y, Sato H, Yamada T, Nagasaki H, Tsuchiya A, Abe R, Yuasa Y: Germ-line mutation of the hMSH6/GTBP gene in an atypical hereditary nonpolyposis colorectal cancer kindred. Cancer Res 1997;57:3920–3923.
48 Kane MF, Loda M, Gaida GM, et al: Methylation of the hMLH1 promoter correlates with lack of expression of hMLH1 in sporadic colon tumors and mismatch repair-defective human tumor cell lines. Cancer Res 1997;57:808–811.
49 Veigl ML, Kasturi L, Olechnowicz J, et al: Biallelic inactivation of hMLH1 by epigenetic silencing a novel mechanism causing human MSI cancers. Proc Natl Acad Sci USA 1998,95: 8698–8702.
50 Herman JG, Umar A, Polyak K, et al: Incidence and functional consequences of hMLH1 promoter hypermethylation in colorectal carcinoma. Proc Natl Acad Sci USA 1998;95:6870–6875.
51 Thibodeau SN, French AJ, Cunningham JM, et al: Microsatellite instability in colorectal cancer: different mutator phenotypes and the principle involvement of hMLH1. Cancer Res 1998;58:1713–1718.

52 Percesepe A, Pedroni M, Sala E, et al: Genomic instability and target gene mutations in colon cancer with different degrees of allelic shifts. Genes Chrom Cancer 2000;27:424–429.
53 Olschwang S, Hamelin R, Laurent-Puig P, et al: Alternative genetic pathways in colorectal carcinogenesis. Proc Natl Acad Sci USA 1997;94: 12122–12127.
54 Salahshor S, Kressner U, Pahlmann L, et al: Colorectal cancer with and without microsatellite instability involves different genes. Genes Chrom Cancer 1999;26:247–252.
55 Järvinen HJ, Mecklin JP, Sistonen P: Screening reduces colorectal cancer rate in families with hereditary nonpolyposis colorectal cancer. Gastroenterol 1995,108:1405–1411.
56 Vasen HF, Nagengast FM, Khan PM: Interval cancers in hereditary non-polyposis colorectal cancer. Lancet 1995;345:1183–1184.
57 Souza RF, Appel R, Yin J, et al: Microsatellite instability in the insulin-like growth factor II receptor gene in gastrointestinal tumors. Nat Genet 1996;14:255–257.
58 Rampino N, Yamamoto H, Ionov Y, et al: Somatic frameshift mutations in the BAX gene in colon cancers of the microsatellite mutator phenotype. Science 1997;275:967–969.
59 Duval A, Gayet J, Zhou XP, et al: Frequent frameshift mutations of the TCF-4 gene in colorectal cancers with microsatellite instability. Cancer Res 1999;59:4213–4215.
60 Sobrero AF, Aschele C and Bertino JR: Fluorouracil in colorectal cancer – a tale of two drugs: implications for biochemical modulation. J Clin Oncol 1997;15:368–381.
61 Lowe SW, Bodis S, McClatchey A, Remington L, Ruley HE, Fisher DE, Housman DE, Jacks T: p53 status and the efficacy of cancer therapy in vivo. Science 1994;266(5186):807–810.
62 Bunz F, Hwang PM, Torrance C, Waldman T, Zhang Y, Dillehay L, Williams J, Lengauer C, Kinzler KW, Vogelstein B: Disruption of p53 in human cancer cells alters the responses to therapeutic agents. J Clin Invest. 1999;104(3): 263–269.
63 Hwang PM, Bunz F, Yu J, Rago C, Chan TA, Murphy MP, Kelso GF, Smith RA, Kinzler KW, Vogelstein B: Ferredoxin reductase affects p53-dependent, 5-fluorouracil-induced apoptosis in colorectal cancer cells. Nat Med 2001;7(10):1111–1117.
64 Arango D, Corner GA, Wadler S, Catalano PJ, Augenlicht LH: c-myc/p53 interaction determines sensitivity of human colon carcinoma cells to 5-fluorouracil in vitro and in vivo. Cancer Res 2001;61:4910–4915.
65 O'Connor PM, Jackman J, Bae I, Myers TG, Fan S, Mutoh M, Scudiero DA, Monks A, Sausville EA, Weinstein JN, Friend S, Fornace AJ Jr, Kohn KW: Characterization of the p53 tumor suppressor pathway in cell lines of the National Cancer Institute anticancer drug screen and correlations with the growth-inhibitory potency of 123 anticancer agents. Cancer Res 1997;57(19):4285–4300.
66 Ahnen DJ, Feigl P, Quan G, Fenoglio-Preiser C, Lovato LC, Bunn PA Jr, Stemmerman G, Wells JD, Macdonald JS, Meyskens FL Jr: Ki-ras mutation and p53 overexpression predict the clinical behavior of colorectal cancer: a Southwest Oncology Group study. Cancer Res 1998;58(6):1149–1158.
67 Goh HS, Yao J, Smith DR: p53 point mutation and survival in colorectal cancer patients. Cancer Res 1995;55(22):5217–5221.
68 Benhattar J, Cerottini JP, Saraga E, Metthez G, Givel JC: p53 mutations as a possible predictor of response to chemotherapy in metastatic colorectal carcinomas. Int J Cancer 1996;69(3): 190–192.
69 Elsaleh H, Powell B, McCaul K, Grieu F, Grant R, Joseph D, Iacopetta B: p53 alteration and microsatellite instability have predictive value for survival benefit from chemotherapy in stage III colorectal carcinoma. Clin Cancer Res 2001;7(5):1343–1349.
70 Watanabe T, Wu TT, Catalano PJ, Ueki T, Satriano R, Haller DG, Benson AB 3rd, Hamilton SR: Molecular predictors of survival after adjuvant chemotherapy for colon cancer. N Engl J Med 2001;344(16):1196–1206.
71 Loehrer PJ Sr, Turner S, Kubilis P, Hui S, Correa J, Ansari R, Stephens D, Woodburn R, Meyer S: A prospective randomized trial of fluorouracil versus fluorouracil plus cisplatin in the treatment of metastatic colorectal cancer: a Hoosier Oncology Group trial. J Clin Oncol 1988;6(4):642–648.
72 Kemeny N, Israel K, Niedzwiecki D, Chapman D, Botet J, Minsky B, Vinciguerra V, Rosenbluth R, Bosselli B, Cochran C, et al: Randomized study of continuous infusion fluorouracil versus fluorouracil plus cisplatin in patients with metastatic colorectal cancer. J Clin Oncol 1990;8(2):313–318.
73 Fink D, Nebel S, Aebi S, Zheng H, Cenni B, Nehme A, Christen RD, Howell SB: The role of DNA mismatch repair in platinum drug resistance. Cancer Res 1996;56(21):4881–4886.
74 Lin X, Howell SB: Effect of loss of DNA mismatch repair on development of topotecan-, gemcitabine-, and paclitaxel-resistant variants after exposure to cisplatin. Mol Pharmacol 1999;56(2):390–395.
75 Lin X, Kim HK, Howell SB: The role of DNA mismatch repair in cisplatin mutagenicity. J Inorg Biochem 1999;77(1–2):89–93.
76 Fink D, Aebi S, Howell SB: The role of DNA mismatch repair in drug resistance. Clin Cancer Res 1998;4(1):1–6.
77 Nehme A, Baskaran R, Aebi S, Fink D, Nebel S, Cenni B, Wang JY, Howell SB, Christen RD: Differential induction of c-Jun NH2-terminal kinase and c-Abl kinase in DNA mismatch repair-proficient and -deficient cells exposed to cisplatin. Cancer Res 1997;57(15):3253–3257.
78 Fink D, Zheng H, Nebel S, Norris PS, Aebi S, Lin TP, Nehme A, Christen RD, Haas M, MacLeod CL, Howell SB: In vitro and in vivo resistance to cisplatin in cells that have lost DNA mismatch repair. Cancer Res 1997; 57(10):1841–1845.
79 Fan S, Smith ML, Rivet DJ 2nd, Duba D, Zhan Q, Kohn KW, Fornace AJ Jr, O'Connor PM: Disruption of p53 function sensitizes breast cancer MCF-7 cells to cisplatin and pentoxifylline. Cancer Res 1995;55(8):1649–1654.
80 Hawkins DS, Demers GW, Galloway DA: Inactivation of p53 enhances sensitivity to multiple chemotherapeutic agents. Cancer Res 1996;56(4):892–898.
81 Smith ML, Ford JM, Hollander MC, Bortnick RA, Amundson SA, Seo YR, Deng CX, Hanawalt PC, Fornace AJ Jr: p53-mediated DNA repair responses to UV radiation: studies of mouse cells lacking p53, p21, and/or gadd45 genes. Mol Cell Biol 2000;20(10):3705–3714.
82 Armand JP, Boige V, Raymond E, Fizazi K, Faivre S, Ducreux M: Oxaliplatin in colorectal cancer: an overview. Semin Oncol 2000;27 (5 suppl 10):96–104.
83 Vaisman A, Varchenko M, Umar A, Kunkel TA, Risinger JI, Barrett JC, Hamilton TC, Chaney SG: The role of hMLH1, hMSH3, and hMSH6 defects in cisplatin and oxaliplatin resistance: correlation with replicative bypass of platinum-DNA adducts. Cancer Res 1998; 58(16):3579–3585.
84 de Gramont A, Vignoud J, Tournigand C, Louvet C, Andre T, Varette C, Raymond E, Moreau S, Le Bail N, Krulik M: Oxaliplatin with high-dose leucovorin and 5-fluorouracil 48-hour continuous infusion in pretreated metastatic colorectal cancer. Eur J Cancer 1997; 33(2):214–219.
85 Fink D, Nebel S, Norris PS, Baergen RN, Wilczynski SP, Costa MJ, et al: Enrichment for DNA mismatch repair-deficient cells during treatment with cisplatin. Int J Cancer 1998;77: 741–744.
86 Giacchetti S, Perpoint B, Zidani R, Le Bail N, Faggiuolo R, Focan C, Chollet P, Llory JF, Letourneau Y, Coudert B, Bertheaut-Cvitkovic F, Larregain-Fournier D, Le Rol A, Walter S, Adam R, Misset JL, Levi F: Phase III multicenter randomized trial of oxaliplatin added to chronomodulated fluorouracil-leucovorin as first-line treatment of metastatic colorectal cancer. J Clin Oncol 2000;18(1):136–147.

Review Article

Digestive Diseases

Dig Dis 2002;20:81–90

Molecular Targets for Prevention of Hepatocellular Carcinoma

Hubert E. Blum

Department of Medicine II, University Hospital Freiburg, Germany

Key Words

HCC primary prevention · HCC secondary prevention · Molecular hepatocarcinogenesis · Chronic liver diseases · HCC epidemiology · HCC natural course · HCC treatment

Abstract

Hepatocellular carcinoma (HCC) is one of the most common malignant tumors in some areas of the world with an extremely poor prognosis. The major etiologic risk factors for HCC development include toxins (alcohol, aflatoxin B1), androgens and estrogens, hepatitis B virus (HBV) and hepatitis C virus (HCV) infection as well as various inherited metabolic disorders, such as alpha-1-antitrypsin deficiency and hemochromatosis. The molecular pathogenesis of HCC development is very complex and involves alterations in the structure or expression of several tumor suppressor genes, oncogenes and, possibly, mechanisms leading to a genetic instability due to mismatch repair deficiency or chromosomal instability and aneuploidy due to defective chromosomal segregation. Central to the molecular pathogenesis of HCCs are mutations of various genes and a genetic instability which in most cases result from chronic liver disease and the associated enhanced liver cell regeneration and mitotic activity. The prognosis of HCC patients is generally very poor. Most studies report a five year survival rate of less than 5% in symptomatic HCC patients. Furthermore, these tumors have been shown to be quite resistant to radio- or chemotherapy. Investigations of the natural history and clinical course of HCCs revealed long-term survival of patients only with small asymptomatic HCCs that could be treated surgically or by non-surgical interventions. Apart from exploring and refining new HCC treatment strategies, the implementation of existing and the development of novel measures to prevent HCC development are most important. Primary HCC prevention includes among others universal hepatitis B vaccination, antiviral therapy of patients with chronic hepatitis B or C, reduction of food contamination with aflatoxins, elimination of excessive alcohol etc. Also for some genetic diseases there is the potential for HCC prevention by identifying affected family members at risk, such as patients with precirrhotic hemochromatosis. Reduction of iron overload by phlebotomy has been shown to eliminate the progression hemochromatosis to liver cirrhosis and HCC. Preventive measures, therefore, should have a major impact on the incidence of HCCs in patients with acquired and inherited liver diseases. Further, the prevention of a local recurrence or the development of new HCC lesions in patients after successful surgical or non-surgical HCC treatment (secondary prevention) is of paramount importance and is expected to significantly

KARGER

Fax + 41 61 306 12 34
E-Mail karger@karger.ch
www.karger.com

0257–2753/02/0201–0081$18.50/0

Accessible online at:
www.karger.com/journals/ddi

Hubert E. Blum, MD
Department of Medicine II, University of Freiburg
Hugstetter Strasse 55
D–79106 Freiburg (Germany)
Tel. +49 761 270 3403, Fax +49 761 270 3610, E-Mail heblum@ukl.uni-freiburg.de

improve disease-free and overall patient survival. Based on rapid scientific advances, molecular diagnosis, gene therapy and molecular prevention are becoming increasingly part of our patient management and will eventually complement and in part replace existing diagnostic, therapeutic and preventive strategies. Overall, this should result in a reduction of the incidence of HCCs, one of the most devastating malignancies worldwide.

Introduction

Hepatocellular carcinoma (HCC) is one of the most common tumors in the world with an estimated 500,000 to 1,000,000 new cases per year. [1] Although less frequent in the United States and Europe, these tumors have an annual incidence of up to 500 cases per 100,000 population in certain regions of Asia and sub-Saharan Africa. The reasons for this high incidence are chronic infections with the hepatitis B virus (HBV) or the hepatitis C virus (HCV) as well as HBV-HCV coinfections [2–9]. The clinical course of HBV and HCV infection depends in part on molecular characteristics of the viruses [10], in part on the patients' HLA haplotype [11–14], in part on other coexisting risk factors. Well recognized non-viral exogenous agents associated with the pathogenesis of HCCs are alcohol and aflatoxins. In the West, alcohol induced liver injury is a leading cause of liver cirrhosis and the most important HCC risk factor [15]. In southern China and Africa, dietary ingestion of high levels of aflatoxin B1 (AFB1) may represent a special environmental hazard, particularly in chronic HBV carriers [16–19]. Other exogenous factors have also been incriminated and include dietary iron overload [20], long-term use of oral contraceptives [21, 22], and high-dose anabolic steroids. The development of liver cirrhosis, particularly in association with genetic diseases, such as alpha-1-antitrypsin deficiency or hemochromatosis, place the individual at a greatly increased risk for the malignant transformation of hepatocytes.

The major clinical risk factor for HCC development is liver cirrhosis since 70–90% of HCCs develop in a macronodular cirrhosis. The HCC risk in patients with liver cirrhosis depends on the activity, duration and the etiology of the underlying liver disease (fig. 1). In addition, HCCs are more frequent in males than in females and the incidence generally increases with age also in the Western world [23–27].

The prognosis of patients with inoperable HCCs is very poor, the patient's estrogen receptor status being the strongest prognostic factor for survival [28]. Unfortunately, despite progress in early diagnosis and surgical as well non-surgical treatment strategies, the overall survival of HCC patients has not significantly improved during the last two decades [29]. Preventive strategies, therefore, are of paramount importance and need to be actively explored in order to reduce the incidence of HCCs. In the following we will discuss some targets for the prevention of HCCs.

Molecular Hepatocarcinogenesis

Central to the concept of molecular carcinogenesis are mutations of oncogenes and tumor suppressor genes as well as genetic instability of cellular DNA, including mismatch repair deficiency and impaired chromosomal segregation [30–34]. In hepatocarcinogenesis, these genetic events occur in the setting of liver cell injury and necrosis associated with an increased rate of hepatocyte regeneration and mitosis. Any exogenous agent, viral or other, that contributes to chronic low-grade liver cell damage and mitosis potentially increases the risk of HCC development, rendering liver cell DNA susceptible to additional genetic alterations. Overall, there are a variety of molecular mechanisms by which environmental and viral carcinogens may play a role in HCC development [35–37].

Oncogenes

Activated cellular oncogenes, particularly those of the *ras* family, have been found in a number of experimental hepatocarcinogenesis models. In human hepatocarcinogenesis, however, no consistent pattern of protooncogene activation has emerged so far for HCC. It is also of interest that no structural or functional changes of a large panel of oncogenes have been found in a transgenic mouse model which is believed to resemble the process of human hepatocarcinogenesis.

Tumor Suppressor Genes

Restriction fragment length polymorphism studies of paired HCC and non-tumorous liver samples have revealed relatively frequent (>20% in ≥10 informative cases) chromosomal allelic losses (loss of heterozygosity, LOH) in HCC on chromosomes 4, 5q, 8p, 10q, 11p, 13q, 16, 16p and 16q, 17p, and 22q suggesting that these sites may harbor tumor suppressor genes involved in the pathogenesis of HCCs. In general, these genetic alter-

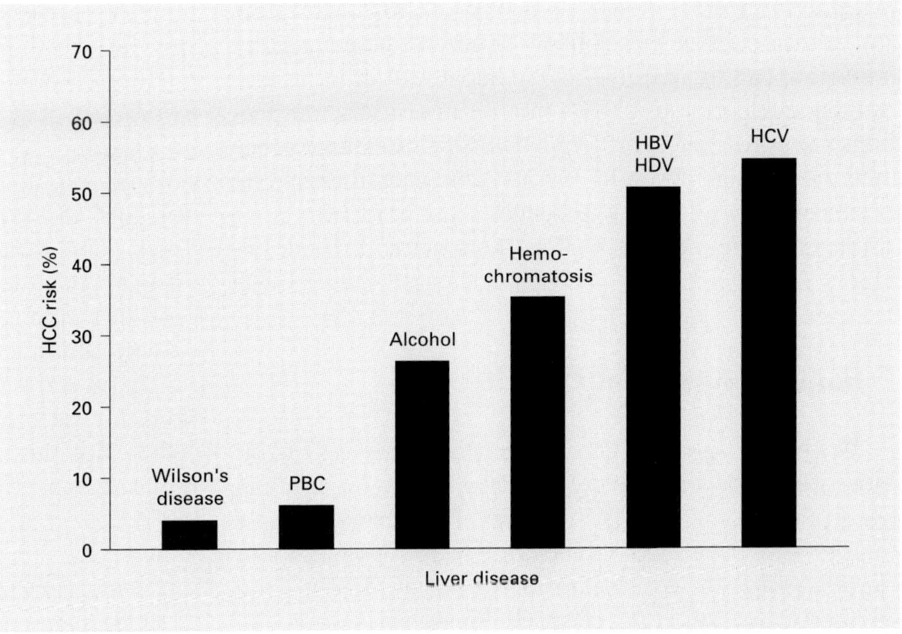

Fig. 1. HCC risk for chronic liver diseases of different etiologies.

ations appear to occur at later stages of HCC development.

Interestingly, a G to T mutation at the third base position of codon 249 of the p53 gene, leading to a substitution of arginine to serine, was found in a significant number of HCCs in patients from southern Africa and the Qidong area in China. It was suggested that this 'hot spot' mutation was associated with high AFB1 intake in food and may have contributed to the high incidence of HCCs in these areas. This finding was supported by in vitro studies indicating that the third base of codon 249 of p53 was preferentially targeted to form adducts with AFB1.

DNA Mismatch Repair Genes

In addition to oncogenes and tumor suppressor genes, DNA mismatch repair genes have recently been identified as a new class of susceptibility genes involved in the pathogenesis of inherited and sporadic human tumors, most notably hereditary nonpolyposis colorectal cancer (HNPCC) [32]. Defective DNA mismatch repair can lead to the accumulation of mutations and microsatellite instability in the cellular genome and thus increase the chance of malignant transformation. The role of DNA mismatch repair defects in HCC development is currently unknown. Recent observations, however, suggest that the hepatitis Bx gene (HBx) may interfere with components of the DNA repair machinery [38].

Telomerase Activation

The progressive shortening of chromosome ends, or telomeres, accompanies normal cell division and may contribute to cellular aging and serve as a control mechanism against unregulated cellular proliferation. Recently, a remarkable correlation between certain types of cancer and the expression of telomerase, a ribonucleoprotein enzyme preventing the shortening of telomeres, was found. Indeed, expression of telomerase may be a common pathway leading to cancer. In this regard, in a recent study telomerase activity was found in 85% of HCC tissues.

Growth Factors

As in most other forms of cancer, the unregulated expression of growth factors and of components of their signalling pathways may play an important role in hepatic oncogenesis. Indeed, overexpression of certain growth factors was found in HCCs, including insulin-like growth factor II, transforming growth factor, hepatocyte growth factor (HGF), and insulin receptor substrate 1. Surprisingly, HGF has been shown to inhibit the growth of a number of hepatoma cell lines and no neoplasms developed in transgenic mice expressing HGF in the liver under control of the albumin promoter. Moreover, in a recent study in c-*myc*-HGF double-transgenic mice it was found that coexpression of HGF markedly reduced c-*myc*-induced neoplastic changes. The knowledge regarding growth factors in HCC, however, is still incomplete and additional factors are likely to emerge as potentially important candidates involved in hepatocarcinogenesis.

Oligonucleotide or cDNA microarray expression profiling, suppression subtractive hybridization and other methods should allow to further elucidate the genetic events underlying HCC pathogenesis and to identify novel diagnostic markers as well as therapeutic targets [39–41].

Natural Course of HCCs

The prognosis of HCC patients is generally very poor. Most studies report a five year survival rate of less than 5% in symptomatic HCC patients. Furthermore, these tumors have been shown to be quite resistant to radio- or chemotherapy. Investigations of the natural history and clinical course of HCC revealed long-term survival of patients only with small asymptomatic HCCs that could be treated surgically or by non-surgical interventions [42]. Most patients (>80%) are inoperable at the time of diagnosis. The prognosis of patients with inoperable HCCs is very poor, the patient's estrogen receptor status being the strongest prognostic factor for survival [28]. Unfortunately, despite progress in early diagnosis and surgical as well as non-surgical treatment strategies, the overall survival of HCC patients has not significantly improved during the last two decades [29]. Preventive strategies, therefore, are of paramount importance and need to be actively explored in order to reduce the incidence of HCCs.

Molecular Therapy of HCCs

Treatment strategies for HCCs include surgical and non-surgical interventions. Gene therapy for HCCs is also being explored in vitro as well as in preclinical models and involves three concepts: gene substitution, gene augmentation and DNA vaccination [43, 44].

Gene Substitution

One of the most intriguing concepts of gene therapy for cancer is restoration of tumor suppressor functions [45], for example by introduction of the wild-type p53 tumor suppressor gene into tumor cells by various gene transfer strategies. Mutations of the p53 tumor suppressor gene are frequently found in HCCs, especially in geographic regions where HBV infection and exposure to AFBI are risk factors [37, 46–49]. Loss of wild-type p53 protein function is associated with the malignant phenotype via a specific growth or survival advantage for liver cells carrying the p53 mutation and enhances the cellular resistance to a variety of chemotherapeutic drugs [50, 51]. Conversely, introduction of a wild-type p53 gene into HCC cells carrying a mutated p53 gene may result in growth inhibition and restoration of sensitivity to chemotherapeutic drugs. This strategy has been successfully explored in vitro by retrovirus mediated transfer of wild-type p53 gene into human HCC cells, resulting in tissue-specific growth inhibition and chemosensitivity to cisplatin [52]. Furthermore, a new and elegant approach uses p53 mutations for selective, adenovirus-mediated lysis of tumor cells. Thus, an adenovirus mutant was engineered that replicates selectively in p53-deficient human tumor cells [53–55].

Gene Augmentation

Gene augmenation is aimed at the local expression of a therapeutic gene product that is physiologically not expressed or expressed at therapeutically insufficient levels. Apart from the expression of cytokines, e.g., interleukin-2 (IL-2) or tumor necrosis factor-alpha (TNF-alpha) the therapeutic principle may be a 'suicide gene'.

Complete regression of a murine HCC has been demonstrated in vivo by TNF-alpha [56], by IL-2 [57] as well as by an activatable interferon regulatory factor-1 in mice [58]. Gene transfer was achieved in vivo by delivering retroviral [56] or adenoviral vectors [57] systemically, directly into the tumor or into the peritoneal cavity. In principle, gene transfer can also be performed ex vivo [59] by transducing tumor infiltrating lymphocytes (TILs) from the patient's HCC with the therapeutic gene, expanding the TILs in vitro and giving the ex vivo modified TILs back to the patient.

Another strategy to treat HCCs is genetic prodrug activation therapy via the introduction of a 'suicide gene' into malignant cells followed by the administration of the prodrug. This concept has been experimentally explored in HCC cells in vitro and in vivo, e.g., for the herpes simplex virus thymidine kinase (HSV-tk) gene [60–64], the gene encoding cytosine deaminase (CD) that converts the prodrug 5-fluorocytosine to 5-fluorouracil which inhibits RNA and DNA synthesis during the S-phase of the cell cycle [65], the gene encoding purine nucleoside phosphorylase that converts purine analogs into freely diffusible toxic metabolites [66, 67] as well as by the gene encoding cytochrome p450 4B1 [68]. A significant bystander effect of cell killing caused by suicide gene expression could be demonstrated in vitro and in vivo, based on cell-cell contact rather than release of cytotoxic substances from the transduced cells [69]. At the same time, the bystander effect may also affect non-malignant dividing cells in the target tissue, potentially limiting the application of this strategy.

DNA Vaccination

An elegant and innovative application of gene therapy is the manipulation of the immune system by introduction of expression vectors into muscle cells, resulting in long-lasting cellular and humoral immune responses [70–73]. DNA-based tumor vaccination against HCC may be possible, for example, by intramuscular introduction of a plasmid expressing HCC-specific antigens or antigens that are highly overexpressed in HCC cells, such as AF-20 antigen, insulin receptor substrate-1 [74], alpha-fetoprotein [75], aspartyl asparaginyl hydroxylase, mutated p53 protein and others. Potential limitations of this strategy include the regulation of the immune response as well as the low level expression of the targeted antigen in non-malignant cells [76], rendering them susceptible to immune-mediated elimination as well.

HCC Prevention

HCC prevention falls into two categories. Primary prevention that is aimed at the prevention of HCC development in patients with chronic liver diseases of different etiologies and secondary prevention that is aimed at preventing the recurrence and/or the development of new HCC lesions after successful surgical or non-surgical HCC treatment.

Primary HCC Prevention

Apart from developing and refining novel therapeutic strategies the implementation of measures for the primary or secondary prevention of HCC development are most important. Primary prevention is aimed at the interference with HCC development at four stages (fig. 2).

Stage 1

Interventions at this step are aimed at the prevention of acquired liver diseases. Apart from avoiding liver toxins, including alcohol and certain drugs, or infections with HBV or HCV by hygienic measures, avoiding parenteral exposure to blood, blood products or contaminated needles etc. a prime example is vaccination against HBV

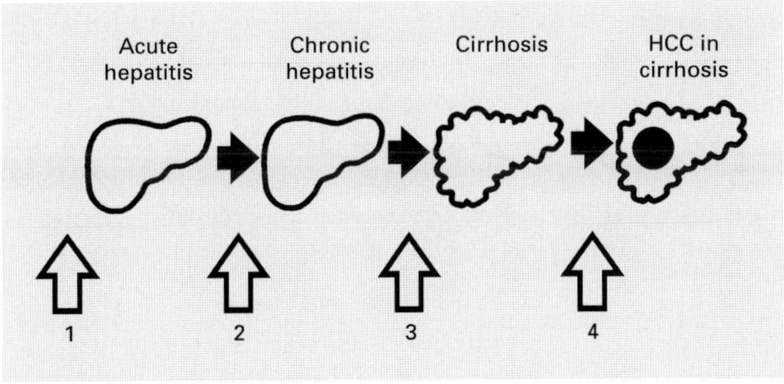

Fig. 2. Primary HCC prevention. 1: Prevention of liver disease, e.g., by hygienic measures, prevention of exposure or vaccination against HBV infection, abstinence from alcohol etc. 2: Prevention of chronic hepatitis; e.g., by treatment of acute hepatitis C, abstinence from alcohol, treatment of hereditary liver diseases etc. 3: Prevention of liver cirrhosis, e.g., by antiviral treatment of chronic hepatitis B or C, treatment of other chronic liver diseases. 4: Prevention of HCC development in liver cirrhosis, e.g., by antiviral treatment, inhibition of fibrosis, liver transplantation etc.

infection using the commercially available active and passive vaccines. Several HBV vaccines using natural or recombinant hepatitis B surface antigen (HBsAg) from different sources are well introduced in clinical practice and universal vaccination in Taiwan has indeed already resulted in a decline of the incidence of HCCs [77]. In addition, novel HBV vaccination strategies are being explored, including a novel triple HBsAg recombinant vaccine [78], epidermal HBsAg powder immunization [79] as well as oral immunization using HBsAg transgenic plants [80–82]. Further, DNA vaccination has been shown in animal models to induce antibodies against HBsAg/anti-HBs [83, 84], even after topical application to the skin. For the prevention of HCV infection, however, there is no effective vaccine available to date. While several HCV vaccination concepts are being evaluated, including HCV proteins [85], HCV-like particles [86] as well as intravenous, intrahepatic, intra-epidermal, intramuscular or oral cDNA immunization [87–91], it is not to be expected that a vaccine against HCV infection will become commercially available within the next few years.

Stage 2

Interventions at this step are aimed at the early treatment of acute liver diseases, thereby blocking their transition into chronic hepatitis that carries the risk for developing liver cirrhosis and its sequelae, including HCC. While the principles mentioned above regarding liver tox-

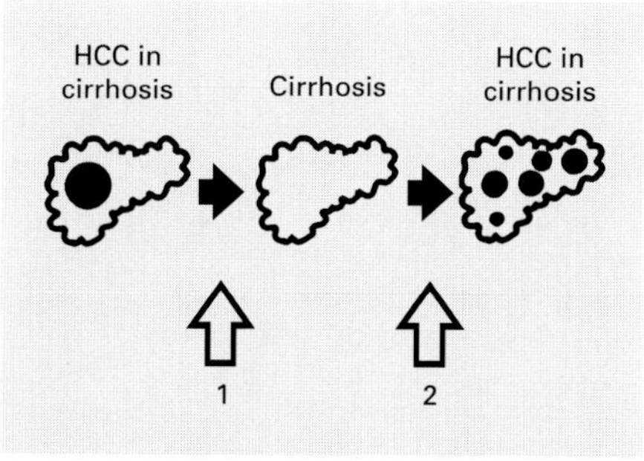

Fig. 3. Secondary HCC prevention. 1: Surgical (resection, liver transplantation) or non-surgical HCC treatment. 2: Prevention of local HCC recurrence or new HCC lesions in cirrhotic liver.

ins also apply here, the early diagnosis and treatment of inherited liver diseases, such as Wilson's disease and hemochromatosis, are of paramount importance. Further, a recent study suggests that early treatment of acute HCV infection prevents its progression to chronic hepatitis C in more than 90% of patients [92].

Stage 3

Interventions at this step are aimed at the prevention of the progression of chronic hepatitis to liver cirrhosis that carries a high risk for HCC development. Apart from avoiding liver toxins or the long-term use of high-dose androgens or other anabolic steroids, the treatment of chronic hepatitis is here most important. This includes the treatment of inherited, cholestatic or autoimmune liver diseases as well as the treatment of chronic viral hepatitis B or C. Reduction of iron overload by phlebotomy, for example, has been shown to stop the progression of hemochromatosis to liver cirrhosis and HCC. Treatment of chronic hepatitis B by interferon alpha or nucleoside analogs [93–95] and chronic hepatitis C by interferon alpha and more recently by its combination with the nucleoside analog ribavirin demonstrated biochemical, virological and histopathologial improvement [96–99] and a lower incidence of HCC development [100–102].

Stage 4

Interventions at this step, other than liver transplantation, are aimed at interfering with the molecular events leading to HCC development, usually in a cirrhotic liver. These strategies include all treatment modalities detailed above (stage 3) as far as they can be implemented in patients with compensated or decompensated liver cirrhosis. In addition, some of the measures to pevent HCC recurrence after successful HCC treatment (secondary prevention, see below) should in principle also be useful for HCC prevention at this stage of the liver disease. Further, some concepts of molecular therapy of HCCs (see above) should be applicable also for the prevention of HCCs. Without experimental pre-clinical data on these issues it would be premature, however, to discuss their potential clinical impact.

Secondary HCC Prevention

The prevention of a local recurrence and/or the development of new HCC lesions in patients after successful surgical or non-surgical HCC treatment (fig. 3) is of paramount importance and is expected to significantly improve disease-free and overall patient survival.

Stage 1

HCC treatment strategies include surgical as well as non-surgical interventions. Surgical interventions are resection and in selected cases liver transplantation [103–106]. Because the majority of patients presents with advanced HCCs at the time of diagnosis or carries a high surgical risk due to comorbidities or advanced age, non-surgical therapeutic interventions are of paramount importance. These include percutaneous ethanol injection (PEI) [107, 108], percutaneous acetic acid injection (PAI) [109], percutaneous thermal ablations, e.g., radiofrequencey thermal ablation (RFTA) [110–112], laser induced thermal ablation (LiTT) [113] as well as transarterial chemotherapy (TAC), transarterial chemoembolisation (TACE) [107, 114] or transarterial iodine-131 lipiodol therapy. In addition, a number of drugs have been evaluated in clinical trials [115, 116]. While tamoxifen and several chemotherapeutic agents has not been shown to be effective in randomized controlled clinical trials, there are a number of substances that deserve further clinical evaluation, e.g., gemcitabine [117, 118], octreotide [119], thymostimulin [120] and pravastatin [121]. Overall, the only potentially curative treatment is surgery, especially liver transplantation. HCC resection and some non-surgical interventions, especially PEI and RFTA, can in selected cases prolong disease-free as well as overall survival with survial rates of about 50% at 5 years and in a few cases even result in long-term remission or cure.

Stage 2

After successful HCC resection or non-surgical ablation, HCC recurrence in the remaining, usually cirrhotic liver is the major limitation of the life expectancy of these patients. The probability of recurrence is about 50% within 3 years after successful treatment [105, 122]. Strategies to prevent HCC recurrence are therefore central to the improvement of survival of HCC patients after initial cure. The strategies explored to date include the administration of polyprenoic acid, an acyclic retinoid [123], of interferon alpha [124] and of interferon beta [125]. Further, adoptive immunotherapy [126] and intraarterial iodine-131 lipiodol treatment [127] has been evaluated in clinical studies. All these interventions have resulted in lower HCC recurrence rates. These findings have to be confirmed, however, in larger randomized controlled studies demonstrating a clear clinical benefit before secondary prevention with one the the strategies mentioned above should enter clinical practice.

Summary and Perspectives

HCC is one of the most common malignant tumors in some areas of the world with an extremely poor prognosis. The major etiologic risk factors for HCC development include toxins (alcohol, AFB1), androgens and estrogens, HBV and HCV infection as well as various inherited metabolic disorders, such as alpha-1-antitrypsin deficiency and hemochromatosis.

The molecular pathogenesis of HCC development is very complex and involves alterations in the structure or expression of several tumor suppressor genes, oncogenes and, possibly, mechanisms leading to a genetic instability due to mismatch repair deficiency or chromosomal instability and aneuploidy due to defective chromosomal segregation. Central to the molecular pathogenesis of HCCs are mutations of various genes and a genetic instability which in most cases result from chronic liver disease and the associated enhanced liver cell regeneration and mitotic activity.

Gene therapy for HCC falls into three categories: gene replacement, gene augmentation and DNA vaccination. In view of the complexity of the genetic events underlying hepatocarcinogenesis, most studies performed to date have focused on gene augmentation as an experimental therapeutic strategy. Despite exciting prospects of nucleic acid-based therapy of HCCs, various delivery, targeting and safety aspects need to be addressed before these concepts will enter clinical practice.

Apart from improving HCC therapy, the refinement and implementation of existing as well as the discovery and development of novel strategies aimed at HCC prevention are most important. Primary prevention has been shown to reduce HCC development in some patient groups at risk. For example, hepatitis B vaccination of children in Taiwan has actually resulted in a decline of the HCC incidence. Further, antiviral therapy of patients with chronic hepatitis B or C should contribute to HCC prevention. Public health measures to reduce food contamination with aflatoxins and to eliminate excessive alcohol use should also reduce the incidence of chronic liver disease, cirrhosis and thereby of HCCs. Apart from primary HCC prevention, interventions aimed at secondary prevention after successful HCC treatment are also a very active area of basic and clinical research. In the future, therefore, preventive measures should have a major impact on reducing the incidence of HCCs, one of the most common and devastating malignancies in the world.

References

1 Schafer DF, Sorrell MF: Hepatocellular carcinoma. Lancet 1999;353:1253–1257.
2 Lee WM: Hepatitis B virus infection. N Engl J Med 1997;337:1733–1745.
3 Di Bisceglie AM: Hepatitis C [see comments]. Lancet 1998;351:351–355.
4 Kew MC, Yu MC, Kedda M-A, Coppin A, Sarkin A, Hodkinson J: The relative roles of hepatitis B and C viruses in the etiology of hepatocellular carcinoma in southern African blacks. Gastroenterology 1997;112:184–187.
5 Donato F, Boffetta P, Puoti M: A meta-analysis of epidemiological studies on the combined effect of hepatitis B and C virus infections in causing hepatocellular carcinoma. Int J Cancer 1998;75:347–354.
6 Okuda K: Hepatocellular carcinomas associated with hepatitis B and C virus infections: Are they any different? Hepatology 1995;22:1883–1885.
7 Lauer GM, Walker BD: Hepatitis C virus infection. N Engl J Med 2001;345:41–52.
8 Di Bisceglie AM: Natural history of hepatitis C: its impact on clinical management. Hepatology 2000;31:1014–1018.
9 Liang TJ, Rehermann B, Seeff LB, Hoofnagle JH: Pathogenesis, natural history, treatment, and prevention of hepatitis C. Ann Intern Med 2000;132:296–305.
10 Blum HE: Variants of hepatitis B, C and D viruses: molecular biology and clinical significance. Digestion 1995;56:85–95.
11 Thursz MR, Kwiatkowski D, Allsopp CE, Greenwood BM, Thomas HC, Hill AV: Association between an MHC class II allele and clearance of hepatitis B virus in the Gambia. N Engl J Med 1995;332:1065–1069.

12 Congia M, Clemente MG, Dessi C, Cucca F, Mazzoleni AP, Frau F, Lampis R, et al: HLA class II genes in chronic hepatitis C virus-infection and associated immunological disorders. Hepatology 1996;24:1338–1341.
13 Tibbs C, Donaldson P, Underhill J, Thomson L, Manabe K, Williams R: Evidence that the HLA DQA1*03 allele confers protection from chronic HCV-infection in northern European caucasoids. Hepatology 1996;24:1342–1345.
14 Kuzushita N, Hayashi N, Moribe T, Katayama K, Kanto T, Nakatani S, Kaneshige T, et al: Influence of HLA haplotypes on the clinical courses of individuals infected with hepatitis C virus. Hepatology 1998;27:240–244.
15 Donato F, Tagger A, Chiesa R, Ribero ML, Tomasoni V, Fasola M, Gelatti U, et al: Hepatitis B and C virus infection, alcohol drinking and hepatocellular carcinoma: a case-control study in Italy. Hepatology 1997;26:579–584.
16 Eaton DL, Gallagher EP: Mechanism of aflatoxin carcinogenesis. Annu Rev Pharmacol Toxicol 1994;34:135–172.
17 Chen C-J, Wang L-Y, Lu S-N, Wu M-H, You S-L, Zhang Y-J, Wang L-W, et al: Elevated aflatoxin exposure and increased risk of hepatocellular carcinoma. Hepatology 1996;24:38–42.
18 Aguilar F, Hussain SP, Cerutti P: Aflatoxin B_1 induces the transversion of GÆT in codon 249 of the p53 tumor suppressor gene in human hepatocytes. Proc Natl Acad Sci USA 1993;90: 8586–8590.
19 Bailey EA, Iyer RS, Stone MP, Harris TM, Essigmann JM: Mutational properties of the primary aflatoxin B_1-DNA adduct. Proc Natl Acad Sci USA 1996;93:1535–1539.
20 Mandishona E, MacPhail AP, Gordeux VR, Kedda M-A, Paterson AC, Rouault TA, Kew MC: Dietary iron overload as a risk factor for hepatocellular carcinoma in black Africans. Hepatology 1998;27:1563–1566.
21 Mant JWF, Vessey MP: Trends in mortality from primary liver cancer in England and Wales. Br J Cancer 1995;72:800–803.
22 Waetjen LE, Grimes DA: Oral contraceptives and primary liver cancer: temporal trends in 3 countries. Obstet Gynecol 1996;88:945–949.
23 Poynard T, Bedossa P, Opolon P, for the METAVIR, CLINIVIR, and, DOSVIRC, et al: Natural history of liver fibrosis progression in patients with chronic hepatitis C. Lancet 1997; 349:825–832.
24 Deuffic S, Poynard T, Buffat L, Valleron A-J: Trends in primary liver cancer. Lancet 1998; 351:214–215.
25 Taylor-Robinson SD, Foster GR, Arora S, Hargreaves S, Thomas HC: Increase in primary liver cancer in the UK, 1979–1994. Lancet 1997; 350:1142–1143.
26 De Vos Irvine H, Goldberg D, Hole DJ, McMenamin J: Trends in primary liver cancer. Lancet 1998;351:215–216.
27 El-Serag HB, Mason AC: Rising incidence of hepatocellular carcinoma in the United States. N Engl J Med 1999;340:745–750.
28 Villa E, Moles A, Ferretti I, Buttafoco P, Grottola A, Del Buono M, De Santis M, et al: Natural history of inoperable hepatocellular carcinoma: estrogen receptors' status in the tumor is the strongest prognostic factor for survival. Hepatology 2000;32:233–238.
29 El-Serag HB, Mason AC, Key C: Trends in survival of patients with hepatocellular carcinoma between 1977 and 1996 in the United States. Hepatology 2001;33:62–65.
30 Fearon ER, Vogelstein B: A genetic model for colorectal tumorigenesis. Cell 1990;61:759–767.
31 Liu B, Nicolaides NC, Markowitz S, Willson JKV, Parsons RE, Jen J, Papadopolous N, et al: Mismatch repair gene defects in sporadic colorectal cancers with microsatellite instability. Nat Genet 1995;9:48–55.
32 Kinzler KW, Vogelstein B: Lessons from hereditary colorectal cancer. Cell 1996;87:159–170.
33 Fearon ER: Human cancer syndromes: clues to the origin and nature of cancer. Science 1997; 278:1043–1050.
34 Kinzler KW, Vogelstein B: Gatekeepers and caretakers. Nature 1997;386:761–763.
35 Moradpour D, Wands JR: The molecular pathogenesis of hepatocellular carcinoma. J Viral Hepat 1994;1:17–31.
36 Moradpour D, Wands JR, Blum HE: Molecular biology of hepatitis B and C virus and hepatocellular carcinoma. Mol Cancer Biol 1996;3: 875–904.
37 Ozturk M: Genetic aspects of hepatocellular carcinogenesis. Semin Liver Dis 1999;19:235–242.
38 Becker S, Lee T-H, Butel J, Slagle B: Hepatitis B virus X protein interferes with cellular DNA repair. J Virol 1998;72:266–272.
39 Miyasaka Y, Enomoto N, Nagayama K, Izumi N, Marumo F, Watanabe M, Sato C: Analysis of differentially expressed genes in human hepatocellular carcinoma using suppression subtractive hybridization. Br J Cancer 2001;85: 228–234.
40 Shirota Y, Kaneko S, Honda M, Kawai HF, Kobayashi K: Identification of differentially expressed genes in hepatocellular carcinoma with cDNA microarrays. Hepatology 2001;33: 832–840.
41 Graveel CR, Jatkoe T, Madore SJ, Holt AL, Farnham PJ: Expression profiling and identification of novel genes in hepatocellular carcinomas. Oncogene 2001;20:2704–2712.
42 Yuen MF, Cheng CC, Lauder IJ, Lam SK, Ooi CG, Lai CL: Early detection of hepatocellular carcinoma increases the chance of treatment: Hong Kong experience. Hepatology 2000;31: 330–335.
43 Blum HE, Linhart HG: Gene therapy for hepatocellular carcinoma. Viral Hepat Rev 1999;5: 147–157.
44 Blum HE, Moradpour D, Köck J, Z.-Y. T, F. vW, W.-B. O: Gene therapy for hepatocellular carcinoma: concepts and perspectives; in W F (ed): Normal and Malignant Liver Cell Growth. Dordrecht, Kluwer, 1999;232–242.
45 Friedmann T: Gene therapy of cancer through restoration of tumor-suppressor functions? Cancer 1992;70:1810–1817.
46 Hsu HC, Chiou TJ, Chen JY, Lee CS, Lee PH, Peng SY: Clonality and clonal evolution of hepatocellular carcinoma with multiple nodules. Hepatology 1991;13:923–928.
47 Scorsone KA, Zhou YZ, Butel JS, Slagle BL: p53 mutations cluster at codon 249 in hepatitis B virus-positive hepatocellular carcinomas from China. Cancer Res 1992;52:1635–1638.
48 Li D, Cao Y, He L, Wang NJ, Gu JR: Aberrations of p53 gene in human hepatocellular carcinoma from China. Carcinogenesis 1993;14: 169–173.
49 Greenblatt MS, Bennett WP, Hollstein M, Harris CC: Mutations in the p53 tumor suppressor gene: clues to cancer etiology and molecular pathogenesis. Cancer Res 1994;54:4855–4878.
50 Lowe SW, Ruley HE, Jacks T, Housman DE: p53-dependent apoptosis modulates the cytotoxicity of anticancer agents. Cell 1993;74: 957–967.
51 Harris CC: Structure and function of the tumor suppressor gene: clues for rational cancer therapeutic strategies. J Natl Cancer Inst 1996;88: 1442–1455.
52 Xu GW, Sun ZT, Forrester K, Wang XW, Coursen J, Harris CC: Tissue-specific growth suppression and chemosensitivity promotion in human hepatocellular carcinoma cells by retroviral-mediated transfer of the wild-type p53 gene. Hepatology 1996;24:1264–1268.
53 Bischoff JR, Kirn DH, Williams A, Heise C, Horn S, Muna M, Ng L, et al: An adenovirus mutant that replicates selectively in p53-deficient human tumor cells. Science 1996;274: 373–375.
54 Heise C, Sampson-Johannes A, Williams A, McCormick F, von Hoff DD, Kirn DH: ONYX-015, an E1B gene-attenuated adenovirus, causes tumor-specific cytolysis and antitumoral efficacy that can be augmented by standard chemotherapeutic agents. Nat Med 1997; 3:639–645.
55 Lowe SW: Progress of the smart bomb cancer virus. Nature Med 1997;3:606–608.
56 Cao G, Kuriyama S, Du P, Sakamoto T, Kong X, Masui K, Qi Z: Complete regression of established murine hepatocellular carcinoma by in vivo tumor necrosis factor alpha gene transfer [see comments]. Gastroenterology 1997;112:501–510.
57 Huang H, Chen SH, Kosai K, Finegold MJ, Woo SL: Gene therapy for hepatocellular carcinoma: long-term remission of primary and metastatic tumors in mice by interleukin-2 gene therapy in vivo. Gene Ther 1996;3:980–987.
58 Kroger A, Ortmann D, Krohne TU, Mohr L, Blum HE, Hauser H, Geissler M: Growth suppression of the hepatocellular carcinoma cell line Hepa1–6 by an activatable interferon regulatory factor-1 in mice. Cancer Res 2001;61: 2609–2617.
59 Ledley FD: Hepatic gene therapy: present and future. Hepatology 1993;18:1263–1273.

60 Ido A, Nakata K, Kato Y, Nakao K, Murata K, Fujita M, Ishii N, et al: Gene therapy for hepatoma cells using a retrovirus vector carrying herpes simplex virus thymidine kinase gene under the control of human alpha-fetoprotein gene promoter. Cancer Res 1995;55:3105–3109.
61 Kaneko S, Hallenbeck P, Kotani T, Nakabayashi H, McGarrity G, Tamaoki T, Anderson WF, et al: Adenovirus-mediated gene therapy of hepatocellular carcinoma using cancer-specific gene expression. Cancer Res 1995;55: 5283–5287.
62 Qian C, Bilbao R, Bruna O, Prieto J: Induction of sensitivity to ganciclovir in human hepatocellular carcinoma cells by adenovirus mediated gene transfer of herpes simplex virus thymidine kinase. Hepatology 1995;22:118–123.
63 Wills KN, Huang WM, Harris MP, Machemer T, Maneval DC, Gregory RJ: Gene therapy for hepatocellular carcinoma: chemosensitivity conferred by adenovirus-mediated transfer of the HSV-1 thymidine kinase gene. Cancer Gene Ther 1995;2:191–197.
64 Kanai F, Shiratori Y, Yoshida Y, Wakimoto H, Hamada H, Kanegae Y, Saito I, et al: Gene therapy for alpha-fetoprotein-producing human hepatoma cells by adenovirus-mediated transfer of the herpes simplex virus thymidine kinase gene. Hepatology 1996;23:1359–1368.
65 Kanai F, Lan KH, Shiratori Y, Tanaka T, Ohashi M, Okudaira T, Yoshida Y, et al: In vivo gene therapy for alpha-fetoprotein-producing hepatocellular carcinoma by adenovirus-mediated transfer of cytosine deaminase gene. Cancer Res 1997;57:461–465.
66 Mohr L, Shankara S, Yoon SK, Krohne TU, Geissler M, Roberts B, Blum HE, et al: Gene therapy of hepatocellular carcinoma in vitro and in vivo in nude mice by adenoviral transfer of the Escherichia coli purine nucleoside phosphorylase gene. Hepatology 2000;31:606–614.
67 Krohne TU, Shankara S, Geissler M, Roberts BL, Wands JR, Blum HE, Mohr L: Mechanisms of cell death induced by suicide genes encoding purine nucleoside phosphorylase and thymidine kinase in human hepatocellular carcinoma cells in vitro. Hepatology 2001;34: 511–518.
68 Mohr L, Rainov NG, Mohr UG, Wands JR: Rabbit cytochrome P450 4B1: A novel prodrug activating gene for pharmacogene therapy of hepatocellular carcinoma. Cancer Gene Ther 2000;7:1008–1014.
69 Kuriyama S, Nakatani T, Masui K, Sakamoto T, Tominaga K, Yoshikawa M, Fukui H, et al: Bystander effect caused by suicide gene expression indicates the feasibility of gene therapy for hepatocellular carcinoma. Hepatology 1995; 22:1838–1846.
70 Wolff JA, Malone RW, Williams P, Chong W, Acsadi G, Jani A, Felgner PL: Direct gene transfer into mouse muscle in vivo. Science 1990;247:1465–1468.
71 McDonnell WM, Askari FK: DNA vaccines. N Engl J Med 1996;334:42–45.
72 Pardoll DM, Beckerleg AM: Exposing the immunology of naked DNA vaccines. Immunity 1995;3:165–169.
73 Donnelly JJ, Ulmer JB, Shiver JW, Liu MA: DNA vaccines. Annu Rev Immunol 1997;15: 617–648.
74 Wands JR, Lavaissiere L, Moradpour D, de la Monte S, Mohr L, Nicolau C, Tanaka S: Immunological approach to hepatocellular carcinoma. J Viral Hepat 1997;4(suppl 2):60–74.
75 Grimm CF, Ortmann D, Mohr L, Michalak S, Krohne TU, Meckel S, Eisele S, et al: Mouse alpha-fetoprotein-specific DNA-based immunotherapy of hepatocellular carcinoma leads to tumor regression in mice. Gastroenterology 2000;119:1104–1112.
76 Geissler M, Mohr L, Weth R, Kohler G, Grimm CF, Krohne TU, von Weizsacker F, et al: Immunotherapy directed against alpha-fetoprotein results in autoimmune liver disease during liver regeneration in mice. Gastroenterology 2001;121:931–939.
77 Chang MH, Chen CJ, Lai MS, Hsu HM, Wu TC, Kong MS, Liang DC, et al: Universal hepatitis B vaccination in Taiwan and the incidence of hepatocellular carcinoma in children. Taiwan Childhood Hepatoma Study Group [see comments]. N Engl J Med 1997;336:1855–1859.
78 Young MD, Schneider DL, Zuckerman AJ, Du W, Dickson B, Maddrey WC: Adult hepatitis B vaccination using a novel triple antigen recombinant vaccine. Hepatology 2001;34:372–376.
79 Chen D, Weis KF, Chu Q, Erickson C, Endres R, Lively CR, Osorio J, et al: Epidermal powder immunization induces both cytotoxic T-lymphocyte and antibody responses to protein antigens of influenza and hepatitis B viruses. J Virol 2001;75:11630–11640.
80 Arntzen CJ: Pharmaceutical foodstuffs – oral immunization with transgenic plants. Nat Med 1998;4:502–503.
81 Kapusta J, Modelska A, Figlerowicz M, Pniewski T, Letellier M, Lisowa O, Yusibov V, et al: A plant-derived edible vaccine against hepatitis B virus. Faseb J 1999;13:1796–1799.
82 Richter LJ, Thanavala Y, Arntzen CJ, Mason HS: Production of hepatitis B surface antigen in transgenic plants for oral immunization. Nat Biotechnol 2000;18:1167–1171.
83 Davis HL, McClusky MJ, Gerin JL, Purcell H: DNA vaccine for hepatitis B: Evidence for immunogenicity in chimpanzees and comparison with other vaccines. Proc Natl Acad Sci USA 1996;93:7213–7218.
84 Prince AM, Whalen R, Brotman B: Successful nucleic acid based immunization of newborn chimpanzees against hepatitis B virus. Vaccine 1997;15:916–919.
85 Choo Q-L, Kuo G, Ralston R, Weiner A, Chien D, van Nest G, Han J, et al: Vaccination of chimpanzees against infection by the hepatitis C virus. Proc Natl Acad Sci USA 1994;91: 1294–1298.
86 Lechmann M, Murata K, Satoi J, Vergalla J, Baumert TF, Liang TJ: Hepatitis C virus-like particles induce virus-specific humoral and cellular immune responses in mice. Hepatology 2001;34:417–423.
87 Lee AY, Manning WC, Arian CL, Polakos NK, Barajas JL, Ulmer JB, Houghton M, et al: Priming of hepatitis C virus-specific cytotoxic T lymphocytes in mice following portal vein injection of a liver-specific plasmid DNA. Hepatology 2000;31:1327–1333.
88 Weiner AJ, Paliard X, Selby MJ, Medina-Selby A, Coit D, Nguyen S, Kansopon J, et al: Intrahepatic genetic inoculation of hepatitis c virus RNA confers cross-protective immunity. J Virol 2001;75:7142–7148.
89 Brinster C, Muguet S, Lone YC, Boucreux D, Renard N, Fournillier A, Lemonnier F, et al: Different hepatitis C virus nonstructural protein 3 (Ns3)-DNA-expressing vaccines induce in HLA-A2.1 transgenic mice stable cytotoxic T lymphocytes that target one major epitope. Hepatology 2001;34:1206–1217.
90 Forns X, Payette PJ, Ma X, Satterfield W, Eder G, Mushahwar IK, Govindarajan S, et al: Vaccination of chimpanzees with plasmid DNA encoding the hepatitis C virus (HCV) envelope E2 protein modified the infection after challenge with homologous monoclonal HCV. Hepatology 2000;32:618–625.
91 Wedemeyer H, Gagneten S, Davis A, Bartenschlager R, Feinstone S, Rehermann B: Oral immunization with HCV-NS3-transformed Salmonella: induction of HCV-specific CTL in a transgenic mouse model. Gastroenterology 2001;121:1158–1166.
92 Jaeckel E, Cornberg M, Wedemeyer H, Santantonio T, Mayer J, Zankel M, Pastore G, et al: Treatment of acute hepatitis C with interferon alfa-2b. N Engl J Med 2001;345:1452–1457.
93 Malik AH, Lee WM: Chronic hepatitis B virus infection: treatment strategies for the next millennium. Ann Intern Med 2001;132:723–731.
94 Torresi J, Locarnini S: Antiviral chemotherapy for the treatment of hepatitis B virus infections. Gastroenterology 2000;118:S83–103.
95 Lok AS, Heathcote EJ, Hoofnagle JH: Management of hepatitis B: 2000 – summary of a workshop. Gastroenterology 2001;120:1828–1853.
96 EASL International Consensus Conference on Hepatitis C. Paris, 26–28, February 1999, Consensus Statement. European Association for the Study of the Liver. J Hepatol 1999;30:956–961.
97 Davis GL: Current therapy for chronic hepatitis C. Gastroenterology 2000;118:S104–114.
98 Manns MP, McHutchison JG, Gordon SC, Rustgi VK, Shiffman M, Reindollar R, Goodman ZD, et al: Peginterferon alfa-2b plus ribavirin compared with interferon alfa-2b plus ribavirin for initial treatment of chronic hepatitis C: a randomised trial. Lancet 2001;358: 958–965.
99 Di Bisceglie AM, McHutchison J, Rice CM: New therapeutic strategies for hepatitis C. Hepatology 2002;35:224–231.

100 Yoshida H, Shiratori Y, Moriyama M, Arakawa Y, Ide T, Sata M, Inoue O, et al: Interferon therapy reduces the risk for hepatocellular carcinoma: national surveillance program of cirrhotic and noncirrhotic patients with chronic hepatitis C in Japan. IHIT Study Group. Inhibition of Hepatocarcinogenesis by Interferon Therapy. Ann Intern Med 1999; 131:174–181.
101 Nishiguchi S, Shiomi S, Nakatani S, Takeda T, Fukuda K, Tamori A, Habu D, et al: Prevention of hepatocellular carcinoma in patients with chronic active hepatitis C and cirrhosis. Lancet 2001;357:196–197.
102 Toyoda H, Kumada T, Nakano S, Takeda I, Sugiyama K, Kiriyama S, Sone Y, et al: Effect of the dose and duration of interferon-alpha therapy on the incidence of hepatocellular carcinoma in noncirrhotic patients with a nonsustained response to interferon for chronic hepatitis C. Oncology 2001;61:134–142.
103 Mazzaferro V, Regalia E, Doci R, Andreola S, Pulvirenti A, Bozzetti F, Montalto F, et al: Liver transplantation for the treatment of small hepatocellular carcinomas in patients with cirrhosis. N Engl J Med 1996;334:693–699.
104 Mor E, Kaspa RT, Sheiner P, Schwartz M: Treatment of hepatocellular carcinoma associated with cirrhosis in the era of liver transplantation. Ann Intern Med 1998;129:643–653.
105 Llovet JM, Fuster J, Bruix J: Intention-to-treat analysis of surgical treatment for early hepatocellular carcinoma: resection versus transplantation. Hepatology 1999;30:1434–1440.
106 Bruix J, Sherman M, Llovet JM, Beaugrand M, Lencioni R, Burroughs AK, Christensen E, et al: Clinical management of hepatocellular carcinoma. Conclusions of the Barcelona-2000 EASL conference. European Association for the Study of the Liver. J Hepatol 2001;35:421–430.
107 Allgaier H-P, Deibert P, Olschewski M, Spamer C, Blum U, Gerok W, Blum HE: Survival benefit of patients with inoperable hepatocellular carcinoma treated by a combination of transarterial chemoembolization and percutaneous ethanol injection – a single-center analysis including 132 patients. Int J Cancer 1998;79:601–605.
108 Yamamoto J, Okada S, Shimada K, Okusaka T, Yamasaki S, Ueno H, Kosuge T: Treatment strategy for small hepatocellular carcinoma: comparison of long-term results after percutaneous ethanol injection therapy and surgical resection. Hepatology 2001;34:707–713.
109 Ohnishi K, Yoshioka H, Ito S, Fujiwara K: Prospective randomized controlled trial comparing percutaneous acetic acid injection and percutaneous ethanol injection for small hepatocellular carcinoma. Hepatology 1998;27: 67–72.
110 Goldberg SN, Gazelle GS, Solbiati L, Livraghi T, Tanabe KK, Hahn PF, Mueller PR: Ablation of liver tumors using percutaneous RF therapy. AJR Am J Roentgenol 1998;170: 1023–1028.
111 Sato M, Watanabe Y, Ueda S, Iseki S, Abe Y, Sato N, Kimura S, et al: Microwave coagulation therapy for hepatocellular carcinoma. Gastroenterology 1996;110:1507–1514.
112 Grasso A, Watkinson AF, Tibballs JM, Burroughs AK: Radiofrequency ablation in the treatment of hepatocellular carcinoma – a clinical viewpoint. J Hepatol 2000;33:667–672.
113 Giorgio A, Tarantino L, de Stefano G, Farella N, Catalano O, Cusati B, Del Viscovo L, et al: Interstitial laser photocoagulation under ultrasound guidance of liver tumors: results in 104 treated patients. Eur J Ultrasound 2000; 11:181–188.
114 Bruix J, Llovet JM, Castells A, Montana X, Bru C, Ayuso MC, Vilana R, et al: Transarterial embolization versus symptomatic treatment in patients with advanced hepatocellular carcinoma: results of a randomized, controlled trial in a single institution. Hepatology 1998;27:1578–1583.
115 Simonetti RG, Liberati A, Angiolini C, Pagliaro L: Treatment of hepatocellular carcinoma: a systematic review of randomized controlled trials. Ann Oncol 1997;8:117–136.
116 Mathurin P, Rixe O, Carbonell N, Bernard B, Cluzel P, Bellin MF, Khayat D, et al: Review article: Overview of medical treatments in unresectable hepatocellular carcinoma – an impossible meta-analysis? Aliment Pharmacol Ther 1998;12:111–126.
117 Yang TS, Lin YC, Chen JS, Wang HM, Wang CH: Phase II study of gemcitabine in patients with advanced hepatocellular carcinoma. Cancer 2000;89:750–756.
118 Kubicka S, Rudolph KL, Tietze MK, Lorenz M, Manns M: Phase II study of systemic gemcitabine chemotherapy for advanced unresectable hepatobiliary carcinomas. Hepatogastroenterology 2001;48:783–789.
119 Kouroumalis E, Skordilis P, Thermos K, Vasilaki A, Moschandrea J, Manousos ON: Treatment of hepatocellular carcinoma with octreotide: a randomised controlled study. Gut 1998;42:442–447.
120 Palmieri G, Biondi E, Morabito A, Rea A, Gravina A, R. BA: Thymostimulin treatment of hepatocellular carcinoma on liver cirrhosis. Int J Oncol 1996;8:827–832.
121 Kawata S, Yamasaki E, Nagase T, Inui Y, Ito N, Matsuda Y, Inada M, et al: Effect of pravastatin on survival in patients with advanced hepatocellular carcinoma. A randomized controlled trial. Br J Cancer 2001;84:886–891.
122 Koike Y, Shiratori Y, Sato S, Obi S, Teratani T, Imamura M, Hamamura K, et al: Risk factors for recurring hepatocellular carcinoma differ according to infected hepatitis virus – an analysis of 236 consecutive patients with a single lesion. Hepatology 2000;32:1216–1223.
123 Muto Y, Moriwaki H, Ninomiya M, Adachi S, Saito A, Takasaki KT, Tanaka T, et al: Prevention of second primary tumors by an acyclic retinoid, polyprenoic acid, in patients with hepatocellular carcinoma. Hepatoma Prevention Study Group. N Engl J Med 1996; 334:1561–1567.
124 Kubo S, Nishiguchi S, Hirohashi K, Tanaka H, Shuto T, Yamazaki O, Shiomi S, et al: Effects of long-term postoperative interferon-alpha therapy on intrahepatic recurrence after resection of hepatitis C virus-related hepatocellular carcinoma. A randomized, controlled trial. Ann Intern Med 2001;134:963–967.
125 Ikeda K, Arase Y, Saitoh S, Kobayashi M, Suzuki Y, Suzuki F, Tsubota A, et al: Interferon beta prevents recurrence of hepatocellular carcinoma after complete resection or ablation of the primary tumor-A prospective randomized study of hepatitis C virus-related liver cancer. Hepatology 2000;32:228–232.
126 Takayama T, Sekine T, Makuuchi M, Yamasaki S, Kosuge T, Yamamoto J, Shimada K, et al: Adoptive immunotherapy to lower post-surgical recurrence rates of hepatocellular carcinoma: a randomised trial. Lancet 2000;356: 802–807.
127 Lau WY, Leung TW, Ho SK, Chan M, Machin D, Lau J, Chan AT, et al: Adjuvant intra-arterial iodine-131-labelled lipiodol for resectable hepatocellular carcinoma: a prospective randomised trial. Lancet 1999;353: 797–801.

Review Article

Digestive Diseases

Dig Dis 2002;20:91–101

The Role of Surgery in the Prevention of Familial Cancer Syndromes of the Gastrointestinal Tract

A. Koliopanos M. Wirtz M.W. Büchler H. Friess

Department of General Surgery, University of Heidelberg, Germany

Key Words

Familial cancers · Gastrointestinal tract · Hereditary non-polyposis colon cancer · Familial adenomatous polyposis · Genetic testing · Endoscopic surveillance · Prophylactic surgery

Abstract

Familial predisposition is a well-recognised risk factor in many gastrointestinal cancers. New developments in molecular genetics may contribute to the identification of cancer-prone families. Recognition of familial clustering and genetic testing can identify other members of the family with a high potential risk for cancer development. Appropriate surveillance mechanisms and management protocols may be initiated in order to prevent cancer and/or to detect cancer at an early stage. In the present article, various types of familial cancer of the gastrointestinal tract are reviewed and surgical, diagnostic and therapeutic issues for the management of esophageal, gastric, colorectal, and pancreatic cancer are emphasized.

Introduction

More than 600 genetic traits are associated with an increased risk of neoplasia [1]. However, the extent to which cancer development risk is attributable to genetic or environmental factors varies among tumor types. Tumors are known to develop as a result of alterations in multiple genes and they progress gradually from normal cells to benign tumors, to dysplastic pre-cancerous lesions, and finally to invasive metastatic cancer. Molecular analysis of inherited cancer susceptibility has shown that germline tumor suppressor gene inactivation, germline oncogene activation, DNA repair defects and ecogenetic traits (i.e. hereditary disorders predisposing to cancer through unusual sensitivity to common carcinogens) are the main mechanisms that are involved in many hereditary cancer syndromes.

Familial clustering of many gastrointestinal cancers is recognised in an increasing number of cases. Therefore, identification of individuals among families with a high potential for cancer development is mandatory for prevention. Tailored diagnostic and therapeutic approaches are necessary for early detection and appropriate anti-cancer treatment. In the present article the role of surgery in diagnostics and treatment of familial gastrointestinal cancer syndromes is reviewed and screening recommendations are emphasized.

KARGER

Fax + 41 61 306 12 34
E-Mail karger@karger.ch
www.karger.com

0257–2753/02/0201–0091$18.50/0

Accessible online at:
www.karger.com/journals/ddi

Helmut Friess, MD
Department of General Surgery, University of Heidelberg
Im Neuenheimer Feld 110, D–69120 Heidelberg
Tel. +49 6221 566900, Fax +49 6221 566903
E-Mail helmut_friess@med.uni-heidelberg.de

Familial Predisposition for Esophageal Squamous Cell Carcinoma

Tylosis is a rare autosomal dominantly inherited syndrome characterized by hyperkeratosis of the skin of the palms and soles and papillomata of the esophagus. Squamous cell carcinomas of the esophagus are common in affected families [2–4]. Therefore, increased surveillance measures by means of upper gastrointestinal endoscopy is strongly recommended in affected families although the rarity of the disorder makes consensus agreement difficult among specialists.

Familial Gastric Cancer

Despite its declining incidence in western countries, gastric cancer remains the second most common cause of cancer death on a world-wide basis and familial clustering occurs in about 10% of the cases [5–7]. Early-onset, histologically poorly differentiated, high grade diffuse gastric cancer has been well described in kindreds carrying a mutation for the calcium-dependent cell-adhesion protein E-cadherin [8–10]. The syndrome represents autosomal dominant inherited susceptibility to gastric cancer with high penetrance (70–80%) and young age of onset (average age 37 years) [11, 12]. Taking into account a 70–80% risk of developing a lethal disease, a prophylactic total gastrectomy should be recommended in those kindred members who test positive for E-cadherin mutations [11–13]. All gastric mucosa should be removed. Although gastric specimens may appear normal by gross pathological examination, microscopic examination often reveals multiple foci of cancer with overlying normal gastric mucosa [12]. Relatives of patients with non-cardia gastric cancer have also been found to have an increased prevalence of gastric atrophy and hypochlorhydria due to *Helicobacter pylori* infection, associated factors which are known to indicate increased risk for gastric cancer development [14–16]. Inasmuch as gastric atrophy and hypochlorhydria to these patients are explained by increased propensity to *H. pylori* infection and not due to its increased prevalence, radical eradication of *H. pylori* infection as well as a close surveillance, preferably with upper gastrointestinal endoscopy, should be considered in subjects from families with non-cardia gastric cancer [17].

Small Intestinal Tumors with Familial Predisposition

Although adenocarcinoma of the small intestine represents 1% of all gastrointestinal tract malignancies including liver, bile ducts and pancreas, it is still the most common malignancy of the small intestine. Patients with Crohn's disease develop adenocarcinomas of the small intestine during the fifth decade of their life after an average of 1.5 decades of disease [18–20]. Tumors are often multicentric and the 2-year mortality rate reaches 80%. It should be mentioned that the differentiation of distal small bowel cancer from Crohn's disease can be extremely difficult without histology [21, 22]. Therefore, close surveillance by means of endoscopy and multiple biopsies are the appropriate approach for patients with Crohn's disease, irrespective of previous operations, because tumors may even arise at ileostomy stomata [23].

Familial Syndrome Associated with Small Intestinal Neoplasms

There are several familial syndromes described which are strong risk factors for intestinal cancer. A synopsis of these syndromes is shown in table 1.

Familial and Hereditary Colorectal Cancer

Approximately 6% all of US citizens will develop colorectal cancer during their lifetime [33]. Colorectal cancer is divided into three categories based on genetic influences: sporadic (approximately 60% of cases), familial (approximately 30% of cases), and hereditary (defined syndromes) [33].

Sporadic colorectal cancer is thought to arise through the adenoma-carcinoma sequence by the accumulation of somatic gene mutations within colon cells in the absence of inherited genetic mutation as an initiating event or a family history of colorectal cancer. The current screening recommendations for average-risk patients include: (a) annual fecal occult blood test after the age of 50 years; (b) flexible sigmoidoscopy every 5 years, and (c) colonoscopy every 10 years or, alternatively, air-contrast barium enema every 5–10 years [34]. When an adenomatous polyp is found the patient should undergo endoscopic or surgical polypectomy and thereafter colonoscopic surveillance every 3 years [35, 36]. In case of colorectal cancer, a colonoscopy should be performed for identification of synchronous lesions, then patients should be treated surgically following current multidisciplinary approach protocols.

Table 1. Synopsis of familial syndromes associated with small intestinal neoplasms

Disease	Characteristics
Bessauds-Hillmand-Augier syndrome	sexual infantilism associated with intestinal polyposis, increased risk of intestinal cancer [24]
Carter-Horsley-Hughes syndrome	diffuse polyposis of the small and large bowel, increased risk of intestinal cancer [25]
Familial adenomatous polyposis	hereditary autosomal dominant trait; intestinal polyposis in association with tumors of ectodermal origin like osteomas, desmoid tumors, epidermoid cysts (Gardner syndrome) or brain tumors (Turcot syndrome)
Cowden's disease/Multiple Hamartoma syndrome	autosomal dominant trait, PTEN gene alterations on chromosome 10q; gastrointestinal polyposis with extented risk of colon, thyroid and breast cancer [26]
Familial juvenile polyposis	autosomal dominant trait, genetic mutations in SMAD4 (DPC4) gene on chromosome 10q; juvenile polyps throughout the gastrointestinal tract, congenital anomalies such as malrotation, hydrocephalus, cardiac lesions etc. familiar predisposition to colorectal, gastric, duodenal, pancreatic cancer [27]
Peutz-Jeghers syndrome	autosomal dominant trait; genetic mutations of the STK11 gene on chromosome 19p; hamartomatous polyps of the gastrointestinal tract, mucocutaneous pigmentation, increased risk of gastrointestinal tumors, pancreatic cancer and benign or malignant genital tumors [28–30]
Ruvalcaba-Myhre-Smith (Bannayan-Zonana) syndrome	autosomal dominant trait; PTEN gene alterations on chromosome 10q; hamartomatous gastrointestinal polyps, dysmorphia, intellectual impairment, gastrointestinal malignancy
Neurofibromatosis Type I (von Recklingshausen's) disease	benign and malignant tumors of the gastrointestinal tract [31, 32]

Familial colorectal cancer refers to a clustering of colorectal cancer cases within the members of a family in the absence of a specific hereditary syndrome. In general, colorectal cancer risk among family members varies with the number of affected relatives and the age at disease onset [37, 38]. Colonoscopy is a safe and effective screening modality, which is used in all prospective studies involving people with a high potential for development of colorectal cancer. Interestingly neoplastic yield from endoscopic screening of families with one or more affected members varies enormously in published series with rates between 10 and 63% for polyp detection and 12 to 22% for the detection of adenomas [39–43]. Patients with first-degree relatives with colorectal cancer or with a first-degree relative with an adenomatous polyp diagnosed at age <60 years should undergo total colonic evaluation, preferably by colonoscopy. Initial colonoscopy should be performed at the age of 40 or 10 years before the age when the youngest affected relative was diagnosed. Patients with a second-degree relative with colorectal cancer or a relative with an adenomatous polyp diagnosed past the age 60 years may be screened as average-risk individuals.

Hereditary non-polyposis colon cancer (HNPCC) refers to the clustering of colorectal cancer cases in families, with the absence of adenomatosis of colon and rectum. The syndrome represents an autosomal dominantly inherited predisposition to various cancers with high penetrance (80–85%) [12, 44–47], and is thought to be caused by an inherited mutation in one of the mismatch repair genes: hMSH2, hMLH1, PMS1, PMS2 or hMSH6 [48–50]. In the Lynch I syndrome colorectal cancer is the only manifestation [51, 52]. However, in the Lynch II syndrome a range of extra-colonic tumors coexist, such as endometrial carcinoma and tumors involving the stomach, small bowel, hepatobiliary tract, pancreas, breast, ovaries, urologic tract, brain, or skin [53–58]. Colorectal cancer is diagnosed at an early age, it is right-sided, multiple and 90% of the cases have microsatellite instability (MSI). In 1990, the International Collaborative Group on HNPCC (hereditary non-polyposis colorectal cancer) established the criteria for the selection of families with HNPCC (Amsterdam criteria). The six criteria are the following: (a) at least 3 relatives should have colorectal cancer; (b) one should be a first-degree relative of the other 2;

(c) at least 2 successive generations should be affected; (d) at least 1 colorectal cancer should be diagnosed before age 50; (e) familial adenomatous polyposis should be excluded, and (f) tumors should be verified by pathological examination. The first step for the recognition of families who might be affected by the syndrome is checking the family history. After this, microsatellite instability and/or a mutation analysis should be conducted depending on the risk level of the family examined. MSI is generally used as a screening tool, which is followed by mutational testing of MSI-positive cases, while MSI-negative cases can be tested on a case-by-case basis [59]. According to the revised HNPCC criteria (Amsterdam II) the range of families at risk for HNPCC have been expanded to those with at least 3 relatives with an HNPCC-associated cancer (colorectal, endometrial, small bowel, ureter or renal pelvis), who meet the aforementioned criteria [60]. The goal of the clinical surveillance and counselling for families with subjects that carry pathologic DNA mismatch repair gene mutations is cancer prevention and/or early detection of precancerous lesions for all the members of the affected family [59].

It should be kept in mind that HNPCC patients get benign tumors at roughly the same rate as the general population, but once an adenoma in the colon or rectum develops it progresses rapidly because of the inherited DNA repair defect [45, 61, 62]. Therefore, early and frequent colonoscopic examination is the preferred surveillance measure [33, 63–66]. A yield of 20% adenomas or early-stage cancers was the result of an early (average age 34 years) and frequent (average interval 3 years) colonoscopic surveillance in 61 members of affected families in Finland, contrasting with the advanced stage of cancer lesions that were detected in the no-surveillance group [66]. Colonoscopy may be started at the age of 25 years and repeated annually thereafter in first-degree relatives of HNPCC patients with confirmed mutation in one of the mismatch repair genes [67]. Endoscopic polypectomy is considered for pedunculated left-sided adenomas while flat, right-sided polyps are commonly surgically excised [59]. The risk of recurrent adenoma or colon cancer should always be taken into consideration for younger patients; the decision of a more aggressive surgical approach such as colectomy should be discussed with the patient at the time adenomas are initially identified [68]. When adenocarcinomas of the colon are encountered a colectomy and ileorectal anastomosis is the surgical treatment to choose. However, total proctocolectomy is the preferred treatment for rectal cancers. Less aggressive surgery should not be performed as metachronous lesions may affect 40% of the patients within 10 years of segmental resection [45, 69, 70]. Moreover, the risk of rectal cancer should always be considered in those cases where subtotal colectomy is performed and annual rectoscopic surveillance may identify new lesions in the remaining rectum [71]. Prophylactic colectomy based upon identified gene mutation in a patient has been discussed but is not fully supported since the life-time risk of colorectal cancer in these individuals is about 80% and not 100% [55, 72].

Although endometrial cancer is second only to colorectal cancer as the most common cancer in HNPCC families, no specific recommendations on surveillance measures exist. Female carriers of appropriate gene mutations should, however, undergo trans-vaginal ultrasound and endometrial aspiration annually beginning at the age of 25 to 35 years. Trans-vaginal ultrasound and CA125 levels have been utilised for screening of ovarian cancer although all the aforementioned methods have their limitations with regard to the early detection of malignancy. Prophylactic hysterectomy with or without oophorectomy should be recommended in those women who have completed their family planning and are operated for colorectal cancer [73].

With respect to other tumors in HNPCC, their infrequency makes the development of consensus on appropriate surveillance difficult. There is no recommended screening for urologic tract cancer. Upper gastrointestinal endoscopy and cytology screening may be initiated at the age of 30 years for members of families that are prone to gastric cancer [67].

Familial adenomatous polyposis (FAP) results from germ-line mutations in the gatekeeper adenomatous polyposis coli (APC) gene on chromosome 5q 21-22 [74]. It represents an autosomal dominant, multisystem disorder which is characterised by hundreds to thousands of adenomatous polyps in the colon and the rectum. The average age when adenomas develop lies within the second decade of life. The average age for colorectal carcinoma is in the fourth decade of life if prophylactic colectomy is not performed. However, the colonic phenotype can vary and in some patients it is referred to as attenuated FAP because only a few polyps may be seen [67]. Extra-colonic manifestations include periampullary adenomas and carcinomas, fundic gland polyps, adenomas and carcinomas of the stomach, papillary carcinomas of the thyroid, hepatoblastomas, osteomas, epidermal cysts, desmoid tumors and medulloblastomas. The life-time risk of developing colorectal cancer is 100%. Therefore, patients with a family history of FAP should undergo endoscopic surveillance beginning at the second decade of their life and it should be repeated every second year. However, along with genetic testing, socio-economic and emotional issues surrounding genetic information on this syndrome have to be taken into account.

Patients with polyposis are candidates for total proctocolectomy and ileoanal anastomosis with or without pouch formation. The ileal pouch procedure, which was introduced 20 years ago, may be done in one, or more frequently, in two stage operations including a temporary ileostomy. It has excellent functional results, a low risk of sexual dysfunction in male patients and a low risk of pouchitis [75–77]. However, the procedure carries a higher risk of postoperative complications and longer recovery than the formerly performed ileorectal anastomosis after subtotal colectomy with rectal preservation [75–80]. Nevertheless, this procedure has gained increasing popularity due to minimal risk of secondary rectal cancer [81–82]. It should be emphasized that the risk for cancer development in the pouch-anal anastomosis still exists and patients with total proctocolectomy and ileal pouch-anal anastomosis should be examined annually by endoscopy [13, 83–85]. A laparoscopic ileo-anal pouch procedure may be performed as well [89].

In selected cases a total colectomy with ileorectal anastomosis may be performed. Predictive factors of risk for secondary cancer are the number, size, and severity of dysplasia of rectal polyps, the location of the pathogenic APC mutation within codons 1250–1500, the length of the rectal stump, the age of the patient and the quality of the endoscopic surveillance after the initial operation [81, 90]. Thus, the procedure is suitable for younger patients with few rectal adenomas and a family history of a mild phenotype. It can also be performed for patients with attenuated FAP, provided that frequent and regular screening rectoscopy will be performed post-surgically [81, 91].

A total abdomino-perineal proctocolectomy and Brooke ileostomy is performed in those patients where rectal removal is necessary for complete adenoma excision.

Two thirds of the polyposis patients also have duodenal adenomas [92–99]. Duodenal or periampullary adenocarcinomas occur in FAP patients at increased incidence in comparison to the general population [100, 101]. Therefore, surveillance of the upper digestive tract might lead to increased life expectancy for these patients if initiated before the age of 30 years. However, the treatment of duodenal adenomas presents some difficult problems. The large number of polyps and their sessile nature make endoscopic identification difficult. Endoscopic removal by means of electrocoagulation and/or laser excision carry a significant risk of scar formation near the periampullary area and of perforation of the duodenal wall [102]. Therefore, surgery is a safe, effective and potentially curative management option although it carries considerable costs. Surgical excision of duodenal polyps through duodenotomy leads to a recurrence within a short time [103]. Partial pancreatoduodenectomy (Whipple procedure) should therefore be an option for large, rapidly growing dysplastic or villous duodenal adenomas (see below). Alternatively, a pancreas-preserving duodenectomy with reinsertion of the pancreatic and common bile duct can be performed.

Ulcerative Colitis

Many studies suggest that genetic factors play a certain role in the pathogenesis of ulcerative colitis. In fact a greater frequency of the disease has been described in family members of patients with confirmed ulcerative colitis [104, 105]. There is an increased risk for the development of colorectal cancer in patients with ulcerative colitis and the incidence of malignancy increases with extended bowel involvement, early age of onset of the disease, severity and duration of the disease. The cumulative incidence of cancer is 5% after 20 years of disease and 12% after 25 years of disease. The chance of developing colorectal cancer for patients who had pancolitis for 30 years increases to 35% [106–111]. Interestingly, patients with ulcerative colitis complicated with sclerosing cholangitis are at increased risk for the development of colorectal cancer [112]. Ulcerative colitis-associated colon cancer is more frequently right-sided and multiple in nature [113, 114]. Therefore, a close endoscopic surveillance is recommended in patients with long-standing colitis. The identification of patients at increased risk for cancer is based on histologically proven dysplasia. Confirmed dysplasia of any grade is an indication for colectomy since the probability of a coexistent carcinoma is relatively high [115]. Total proctocolectomy is the procedure of choice and subtotal colectomy with ileorectal anastomosis should be reserved only for patients who refuse proctectomy. This is recommended due to the increased risk to develop secondary rectal cancer, which may be approximately 15% at 40 years after the operation [116]. End-ileostomy (Brooke) and Kock continent ileostomy with pouch formation have been abandoned today in favour for the ileal pouch ileo-anal anastomotic technique which is usually performed in two stages. The first stage consists of abdominal colectomy, mucosal proctectomy, endorectal ileal pouch-anal anastomosis and diverting loop ileostomy. At the second stage, which is performed eight to twelve weeks after the initial operation, the ileostomy is closed. The postoperative and functional results in most published series are remarkably good although the risk for cancer development in ileal pouch mucosa still exists and patients should therefore be screened after the operation [117]. Finally it should be mentioned that colorectal cancer history in patients with ulcerative colitis represents a risk factor for colorectal cancer in their non-colitic relatives. Accordingly, a family history of sporadic colorectal cancer increases the risk for colorectal cancer in patients with ulcerative colitis [118, 119].

Hereditary Pancreatic Cancer

Inherited syndromes that are associated with an increased risk of pancreatic cancer include: (1) hereditary nonpolyposis colorectal cancer (HNPCC); (2) hereditary chronic pancreatitis; (3) familial adenomatous polyposis (FAP); (4) familial atypical multiple mole melanoma (FAMMM), (5) Peutz-Jeghers syndrome; (6) familial breast cancer associated with BRCA2 mutations; (7) ataxia-telangiectasia syndrome, and (8) cystic fibrosis [120]. It has been determined that germline mutations in the BRCA1, BRCA2, p16, LKB1/STK11 and cationic trypsinogen genes contribute to the inherited forms of pancreatic cancer, the last most likely via hereditary chronic pancreatitis [121–123].

It is accepted that, similar to other tumors, the morphological background for the development of pancreatic carcinoma in patients from hereditary pancreatic cancer (HC) kindreds in dysplasia [124–128]. The need to diagnose pancreatic cancer at an early stage in order to improve prognosis has led to the evolution of different diagnostic modalities [129]. Endoscopic ultrasonography, which is a sensitive and specific technique for the detection of pancreatic adenocarcinomas [130–132] may be used and suspicious lesions include (1) heterogeneous parenchyma with 1 to 2 mm echogenic foci scattered throughout; (2) hyperechoic nodules of 2 to 4 mm size; (3) hyperechoic main duct walls, and (4) distinct masses in the pancreatic parenchyma. However, experience in the detection of dysplasia is still very limited and the difficulty is that similar changes can be seen in patients with chronic pancreatitis [124]. However, endoscopic ultrasonography, when performed by experienced investigators, is a safe procedure and may be completed by fine needle aspiration cytology when focal lesions are detected [133–135].

ERCP should be used only when there are changes in the EUS or in the presence of symptoms (persistent epigastric pain, steatorrhoea, jaundice, diabetes mellitus) [124]. Findings that have thus far been associated with dysplasia are an irregular main duct and sacculations or ectatic side branches.

Computed tomography seems to be ineffective for surveillance of patients with the risk of hereditary pancreatic cancer transformation since findings in CT in the presence of dysplasia could be normal or suggestive of chronic pancreatitis due to the fact that dysplasia is multifocal, doesn't produce a definable mass lesion, and occurs normally in the small and medium-sized pancreatic ducts, without affecting the main pancreatic duct [124, 136]. However, CT should be performed when EUS and ERCP findings are positive.

For other diagnostic modalities such as positron emission tomography and intraductal ultrasonography only very limited experience is available [129, 137–139].

Molecular markers that are sensitive and specific for pancreatic cancer such as K-ras, telomerase, CA19-9, and other 'tumor' markers, lack the sensitivity and specificity needed to identify cancer at an early stage or to accurately diagnose the presence of dysplasia [140–143]. The goal of surveillance of patients with a risk of hereditary pancreatic cancer is to diagnose dysplastic lesions before they develop into invasive cancer, and to proceed to total duodenopancreatectomy. False-positive findings of dysplastic changes will lead to unnecessary early pancreatic surgery with all the associated risks. Although morbidity and mortality rates of total pancreatectomy in centers of pancreatic surgery are low, the resultant diabetes mellitus that the patient will develop is not at all trivial or insignificant.

The Extent of Surgical Intervention

The multifocal nature of dysplastic lesions precludes any type of operation that would preserve pancreatic tissue. In a recent report, atypical papillary hyperplasia was found incidentally in three patients who underwent partial pancreatic resection, all of whom subsequently developed cancer in the remaining pancreas within 17 months, 9 years and 10 years [144]. Inasmuch as pancreatic cancer is frequently associated with intraductal proliferative lesions, it has been postulated that once dysplasia is present in the pancreatic parenchyma, pancreatic cancer will develop, just as there is progression from adenoma to infiltrating carcinoma of the colon. Taking this concept into consideration, prophylactic whole-organ resection seems to be the management of choice. However, multiple frozen pancreatic sections should be obtained intraoperatively, since the diagnosis of dysplasia can only be confirmed histologically, and if dysplasia is absent, the pancreas or part of it can be preserved. In line with this management strategy, in patients with hereditary pancreatic cancer or kindreds of such patients, any pancreatic lesion which is shown in any imaging procedure needs to be carefully evaluated and in case of any doubt on a benign lesion surgery should be performed. Intraoperatively, the decision for head or left resection should then be based on the type and location of the lesion and frozen section analysis of the remaining pancreas. All patients should be followed by imaging procedures in 6 to 12 month intervals after partial pancreatic resection for hereditary pancreatic cancer.

Another possible way to manage patients with an inherited cancer predisposition is prophylactic whole-organ resection at a stage where morphological changes are present, but dysplasia or carcinoma in situ is not obvious. Concerning prophylactic pancreatectomy in high-risk patients, several factors have to be taken into serious consideration: (1) the perioperative morbidity and mortality associated with the operation; (2) the potential for the patient to develop a brittle diabetes mellitus, and (3) the unknown exact risk of developing pancreatic cancer [145, 146]. In these patients, genetic counseling and psychological support are mandatory to help them to cope with the situation, since prophylactic total pancreatectomy is ultimately the decision of the patient.

During the operation it is also important to search for ectopic pancreatic tissue, which can be found in the stomach and the duodenum but can also be found elsewhere [147]. Ectopic pancreas is usually functional and can produce symptoms as well as contains the risk of developing dysplastic changes and malignancy [124].

So far the presentation and prognosis of patients with inherited forms of pancreatic cancer seems to be similar to that of sporadic disease. Therefore these patients should be treated accordingly. Options in the management of familial pancreatic cancer depend on the stage of the disease.

After pancreatic cancer resection, the long-term results are persistently poor due to the biological nature of this malignancy, which exhibits aggressive local invasion and metastasis during early development. Even in small pancreatic tumors which have not spread through the pancreatic capsule, positive para-aortic lymph nodes are present in 40% [148]. However, due to the resistance of pancreatic cancer to radiation and chemotherapy, radical resection represents the only therapy with the potential for cure. The pylorus-preserving Whipple operation may be the procedure of choice for the treatment of pancreatic and periampullary cancers because it allows a near-normal postoperative nutritional state and results in advantages in quality of life for the patient without an increase in morbidity, mortality, radicallity, local tumor control, local recurrence and survival over the classical Whipple operation [149]. For cancer of the body and tail, distal pancreatectomy with splenectomy is the current standard procedure. Other operations that are more radical, like regional pancreatectomy and resection with extended lymph node dissection, have not shown any advantage in long-term survival [150]. Once cancer has reached an advanced tumor stage in a hereditary pancreatic cancer kindred patient, 'prophylactic' total pancretectomy, as would have been performed in the presence of dysplasia, no longer seems advisable, since the patient will most probably die due to recurrence before a new cancer lesion develops in the remaining preserved pancreas. However, if early pancreatic cancer is present and radical tumor resection is possible, total pancreatectomy should be considered in these patients.

Acknowledgement

The authors thank Prof. Dale E. Bockman for correcting the manuscript.

References

1 Online Mendelian Inheritance in Man, OMIM™: The Human Genome Data Base Project. Baltimore, Johns Hopkins University, 1995.

2 Munoz N, Crespi M: High risk conditions and precancerous lesions of the esophagus; in Sherlock P, Morson BC, Barbara L, Veronesi U (eds): Precancerous lesions of the gastrointestinal tract. New York, Raven Press, 1983, p 53.

3 Marger RS, Marger D: Carcinoma of the esophagus and tylosis. A lethal genetic combination. Cancer 1993;72:17–19.

4 Ashworth MT, Nash JR, Ellis A, Day DW: Abnormalities of differentiation and maturation in the oesophageal squamous epithelium of patients with tylosis: Morphological features. Histopathology 1991;19:303–310.

5 Zanghieri G, Di Gregorio C, Sacchetti C, Fante R, Sassatelli R, Cannizzo G, Carriero A, Ponz de Leon M: Familial occurrence of gastric cancer in the 2-year experience of a population-based registry. Cancer 1990;66:2047–2051.

6 Cwern M, Garcia RL, Davidson MI, Friedman IH: Simultaneous occurrence of gastric carcinoma in identical twins. Am J Gastroenterol 1981;75:41–47.

7 Dhillon PK, Farrow DC, Vaughan TL, Chow WH, Risch HA, Gammon MD, Mayne ST, Stanford JL, Schoenberg JB, Ahsan H, Dubrow R, West AB, Rotterdam H, Blot WJ, Fraumeni JF Jr: Family history of cancer and risk of esophageal and gastric cancers in the United States. Int J Cancer 2001;93:148–152.
8 Guilford P, Hopkins J, Harraway J, McLeod M, McLeod N, Harawira P, Taite H, Scoular R, Miller A, Reeve AE: E-cadherin germline mutations in familial gastric cancer. Nature 1998; 392:402–405.
9 Dunbier A, Guilford P: Hereditary diffuse gastric cancer. Adv Cancer Res 2001;83:55–65.
10 Caldas C, Carneiro F, Lynch HT, Yokota J, Wiesner GL, Powell SM, Lewis FR, Huntsman DG, Pharoah PD, Jankowski JA, MacLeod P, Vogelsang H, Keller G, Park KG, Richards FM, Maher ER, Gayther SA, Oliveira C, Grehan N, Wight D, Seruca R, Roviello F, Ponder BA, Jackson CE: Familial gastric cancer: Overview and guidelines for management. J Med Genet 1999;36:873–880.
11 Huntsman DG, Carneiro F, Lewis FR, MacLeod PM, Hayashi A, Monaghan KG, Maung R, Seruca R, Jackson CE, Caldas C: Early gastric cancer in young, asymptomatic carriers of germ-line E-cadherin mutations. N Engl J Med 2001;344:1904–1909.
12 Lewis FR, Mellinger JD, Hayashi A, Lorelli D, Monaghan KG, Carneiro F, Huntsman DG, Jackson CE, Caldas C: Prophylactic total gastrectomy for familial gastric cancer. Surgery 2001;130:612–617; discussion 617–619.
13 Chun YS, Lindor NM, Smyrk TC, Petersen BT, Burgart LJ, Guilford PJ, Donohue JH: Germline E-cadherin gene mutations: Is prophylactic total gastrectomy indicated? Cancer 2001;92:181–187.
14 Correa P, Haenszel W, Cuello C, Tannenbaum S, Archer M: A model for gastric cancer epidemiology. Lancet 1975;ii:58–60.
15 Correa P: Human gastric carcinogenesis: A multistep and multifactorial process – First American Cancer Society Award Lecture on Cancer Epidemiology and Prevention. Cancer Res 1992;52:6735–6740.
16 Haruma K, Yoshihara M, Sumii K, Tari A, Watanabe C, Kodoi A, Kajiyama G: Gastric acid secretion, serum pepsinogen I, and serum gastrin in Japanese with gastric hyperplastic polyps or polypoid-type early gastric carcinoma. Scand J Gastroenterol 1993;28:633–637.
17 El-Omar EM, Oien K, Murray LS, El-Nujumi A, Wirz A, Gillen D, Williams C, Fullarton G, McColl KE: Increased prevalence of precancerous changes in relatives of gastric cancer patients: Critical role of *H. pylori*. Gastroenterology 2000;118:22–30.
18 Hawker PC, Gyde SN, Thompson H, Allan RN: Adenocarcinoma of the small intestine complicating Crohn's disease. Gut 1982;23: 188–193.
19 Frank JD, Shorey BA: Adenocarcinoma of the small bowel as a complication of Crohn's disease. Gut 1973;14:120–124.
20 Michelassi F, Testa G, Pomidor WJ, Lashner BA, Block GE: Adenocarcinoma complicating Crohn's disease. Dis Colon Rectum 1993;36: 654–661.
21 Ribeiro MB, Greenstein AJ, Heimann TM, Yamazaki Y, Aufses AH Jr: Adenocarcinoma of the small intestine in Crohn's disease. Surg Gynecol Obstet 1991;173:343–349.
22 Adler SN, Lyon DT, Sullivan PD: Adenocarcinoma of the small bowel. Clinical features, similarity to regional enteritis, and analysis of 338 documented cases. Am J Gastroenterol 1982; 77:326–330.
23 Mason G: Tumors of the duodenum and small intestine; in Sabiston D (ed): Textbook of Surgery. The biological basis of modern surgical practice, ed 15. Philadelphia, Saunders, 1997, p 884.
24 Ravitsch M: Discussion of 'A new form of diffuse familial polyposis: A probable genetic explanation' by Carter BN 2nd, Horsley GW, Horsley JS 3rd, Hughes RD. Ann Surg 1968; 167:942–948.
25 Carter BN 2nd, Horsley GW, Horsley JS 3rd, Hughes RD: A new form of diffuse familial polyposis: A probable genetic explanation. Ann Surg 1968;167:942–948.
26 Gold BM, Bagla S, Zarrabi MH: Radiologic manifestations of Cowden disease. Am J Roentgenol 1980;135:385–387.
27 Ivanovich JL, Read TE, Ciske DJ, Kodner IJ, Whelan AJ: A practical approach to familial and hereditary colorectal cancer. Am J Med 1999;107:68–77.
28 Giardiello FM, Brensinger JD, Tersmette AC, Goodman SN, Petersen GM, Booker SV, Cruz-Correa M, Offerhaus JA: Very high risk of cancer in familial Peutz-Jeghers syndrome. Gastroenterology 2000;119:1447–1453.
29 Yoon KA, Ku JL, Choi HS, Heo SC, Jeong SY, Park YJ, Kim NK, Kim JC, Jung PM, Park JG: Germline mutations of the STK1 gene in Korean Peutz-Jeghers syndrome patients. Br J Cancer 2000;82:1403–1406.
30 Westerman AM, Entius MM, de Baar E, Boor PP, Koole R, van Velthuysen ML, Offerhaus GJ, Lindhout D, de Rooji FW, Wilson JH: Peutz-Jeghers syndrome: 78-year follow-up of the original family. Lancet 1999;353:1211–1215.
31 Hochberg FH, Dasilva AB, Galdabini J, Richardson EP Jr: Gastrointestinal involvement in von Recklinghausen's neurofibromatosis. Neurology 1974;24:1144–1151.
32 Inai K, Kobuke T, Yonehara S, Tokuoka S: Duodenal gangliocytic paraganglioma with lymph node metastasis in a 7-year-old boy. Cancer 1989;63:2540–2545.
33 Byers T, Levin B, Rothenberger D, Dodd GD, Smith RA: American Cancer Society guidelines for screening and surveillance for early detection of colorectal polyps and cancer (update 1997). American Cancer Society Detection and treatment Advisory Group on Colorectal Cancer. CA Cancer J Clin 1997;47:154–160.
34 Winawer SJ, Fletcher RH, Miller L, Godlee F, Stolar MH, Mulrow CD, Woolf SH, Glick SN, Ganiats TG, Bond JH, Rosen L, Zapka JG, Olsen SJ, Giardiello FM, Sisk JE, Van Antwerp R, Brown-Davis C, Marciniak DA, Mayer RJ: Colorectal cancer screening: Clinical guidelines and rationale. Gastroenterology 1997;112: 594–642.
35 Winawer SJ, Zauber AG, O'Brien MJ, Ho MN, Gottlieb L, Sternberg SS, Waye JD, Bond J, Schapiro M, Stewart ET: Randomized comparison of surveillance intervals after colonoscopic removal of newly diagnosed adenomatous polyps. The National Polyp Study Workgroup. N Engl J Med 1993;328:901–906.
36 Read TE, Read JD, Butterly LF: Importance of adenomas 5 mm or less in diameter that are detected by sigmoidoscopy. N Engl J Med 1997;336:8–12.
37 St John DJ, McDermott FT, Hopper JL, Debney EA, Johnson WR, Hughes ES: Cancer risk in relatives of patients with common colorectal cancer. Ann Intern Med 1993;118:785–790.
38 Slack J: Family cancer syndromes. J R Soc Med 1989;82:233–234.
39 Luchtefeld MA, Syverson D, Solfelt M, MacKeigan JM, Krystosek R, Waller J, Milsom JW: Is colonoscopic screening appropriate in asymptomatic patients with family history of colon cancer? Dis Colon Rectum 1991;34:763–768.
40 Gryska PV, Cohen AM: Screening asymptomatic patients at high risk for colon cancer with full colonoscopy. Dis Colon Rectum 1987;30: 18–20.
41 McConnell JC, Nizin JS, Slade MS: Colonoscopy in patients with a primary family history of colon cancer. Dis Colon Rectum 1990;33:105–107.
42 Orrom WJ, Brzezinski WS, Wiens EW: Hereditary and colorectal cancer. A prospective, community-based, endoscopic study. Dis Colon Rectum 1990;33:490–493.
43 Gaglia P, Atkin WS, Whitelaw S, Talbot IC, Williams CB, Northover JM, Hodgson SV: Variables associated with the risk of colorectal adenomas in asymptomatic patients with a family history of colorectal cancer. Gut 1995; 36:385–390.
44 Marra G, Boland CR: Hereditary nonpolyposis colorectal cancer: The syndrome, the genes, and historical perspectives. J Natl Cancer Inst 1995;87:1114–1125.
45 Lynch HT, Smyrk T, Lynch J: An update of HNPCC (Lynch syndrome). Cancer Genet Cytogenet 1997;93:84–99.
46 Utsunomiya J, Miyaki M: Studies of hereditary nonpolyposis colorectal cancer in Japan. Int J Clin Oncol 1998;353–374.
47 Jass JR: Diagnosis of hereditary non-polyposis colorectal cancer. Histopathology 1998;32: 491–497.
48 Peltomaki P, Vasen HF: Mutations predisposing to hereditary nonpolyposis colorectal cancer: Database and results of collaborative study. The International Collaborative Group on Hereditary Nonpolyposis Colorectal Cancer. Gastroenterology 1997;113:1146–1158.

49 Miyaki M, Konishi M, Tanaka K, Kikuchi-Yanoshita R, Muraoka M, Yasuno M, Igari T, Koike M, Chiba M, Mori T: Germline mutation of MSH6 as the cause of hereditary nonpolyposis colorectal cancer. Nat Genet 1997;17:271–272.
50 Akiyama Y, Sato H, Yamada T, Nagasaki H, Tsuchiya A, Abe R, Yuasa Y: Germ-line mutation of the hMSH6/GTBP gene in an atypical hereditary nonpolyposis colorectal cancer kindred. Cancer Res 1997;57:3920–3923.
51 Lynch HT, Smyrk TC, Watson P, Lanspa SJ, Lynch JF, Lynch PM, Cavalieri RJ, Boland CR: Genetics, natural history, tumor spectrum, and pathology of hereditary nonpolyposis colorectal cancer: An updated review. Gastroenterology 1993;104:1535–1549.
52 Lynch HT, Lynch PM, Pester J, Fusaro RM: The cancer family syndrome. Rare cutaneous phenotypic linkage of Torre's syndrome. Arch Intern Med 1981;141:607–611.
53 Watson P, Lynch HT: Extracolonic cancer in hereditary nonpolyposis colorectal cancer. Cancer 1993;71:677–685.
54 Vasen HF, Offerhaus GJ, den Hartog Jager FC, Menko FH, Nagengast FM, Griffioen G, van Hogezand RB, Heintz AP: The tumour spectrum in hereditary non-polyposis colorectal cancer: A study of 24 kindreds in the Netherlands. Int J Cancer 1990;46:31–34.
55 Vasen HF, Wijnen, JT, Menko FH, Kleibeuker JH, Taal BG, Griffioen G, Nagengast FM, Meijers-Heijboer EH, Bertario L, Varesco L, Bisgaard ML, Mohr J, Fodde R, Khan PM: Cancer risk in families with hereditary nonpolyposis colorectal cancer diagnosed by mutation analysis. Gastroenterology 1996;110:1020–1027.
56 Vasen HF, Sanders EA, Taal BG, Nagengast FM, Griffioen G, Menko FH, Kleibeuker JH, Houwing-Duistermaat JJ, Meera Khan P: The risk of brain tumours in hereditary non-polyposis colorectal cancer (HNPCC). Int J Cancer 1996;65:422–425.
57 Sijmons RH, Kiemeney LA, Witjes JA, Vasen HF: Urinary tract cancer and hereditary nonpolyposis colorectal cancer: Risks and screening options. J Urol 1998;160:466–470.
58 Aarnio M, Mecklin JP, Aaltonen LA, Nystrom-Lahti M, Jarvinen HJ: Life-time risk of different cancers in hereditary non-polyposis colorectal cancer (HNPCC) syndrome. Int J Cancer 1995;64:430–433.
59 Lynch PM: Clinical challenges in management of familial adenomatous polyposis and hereditary nonpolyposis colorectal cancer. Cancer 1999;86:2533–2539.
60 Vasen HF, Watson P, Mecklin JP, Lynch HT: New clinical criteria for hereditary nonpolyposis colorectal cancer (HNPCC, Lynch syndrome) proposed by the International Collaborative group on HNPCC. Gastroenterology 1999;116:1453–1456.
61 Vogelstein B: Genetic testings for cancer: The surgeon's critical role. Familial colon cancer. J Am Coll Surg 1999;188:74–79.
62 Jass JR: Colorectal adenoma progression and genetic change: Is there a link? Ann Med 1995;27:301–306.
63 Lanspa SJ, Lynch HT, Smyrk TC, Strayhorn P, Watson P, Lynch JF, Jenkins JX, Appelman HD: Colorectal adenomas in the Lynch syndromes. Results of a colonoscopy screening program. Gastroenterology 1990;98:1117–1122.
64 Mecklin JP, Jarvinen HJ, Aukee S, Elomaa I, Karjalainen K: Screening for colorectal carcinoma in cancer family syndrome kindreds. Scand J Gastroenterol 1987;22:449–453.
65 Vasen HF, Taal BG, Nagengast FM, Griffioen G, Menko FH, Kleibeuker JH, Offerhaus GJ, Meera Khan P: Hereditary nonpolyposis colorectal cancer: Results of long-term surveillance in 50 families. Eur J Cancer 1995;31:1145–1148.
66 Green SE, Chapman PD, Burn J, Bishop DT, Varma JS: Clinical impact of colonoscopic screening in first-degree relatives of patients with hereditary non-polyposis colorectal cancer. Br J Surg 1995;82:1338–1340.
67 Lynch HT, Smyrk TC: Hereditary colorectal cancer. Semin Oncol 1999;26:478–484.
68 Burke W, Petersen G, Lynch P, Botkin J, Daly M, Garber J, Kahn MJ, McTiernan A, Offit K, Thomson E, Varricchio C: Recommendations for follow-up care of individuals with an inherited predisposition to cancer. I. Hereditary nonpolyposis colon cancer. Cancer Genetics Studies Consortium. JAMA 1997;277:915–919.
69 Lynch HT, Smyrk T: Hereditary nonpolyposis colorectal cancer (Lynch syndrome). An updated review. Cancer 1996;78:1149–1167.
70 Bellacosa A, Genuardi M, Anti M, Viel A, Ponz de Leon M: Hereditary nonpolyposis colorectal cancer: Review of clinical, molecular genetics, and counseling aspects. Am J Med Genet 1996;62:353–364.
71 Rodriguez-Bigas MA, Vasen HF, Pekka-Mecklin J, Myrhoj T, Rozen P, Bertario L, Jarvinen JH, Jass JR, Kunitomo K, Nomizu T, Driscoll DL: Rectal cancer risk in hereditary nonpolyposis colorectal cancer after abdominal colectomy. International Collaborative Group on HNPCC. Ann Surg 1997;225:202–207.
72 Lynch HT: Is there a role for prophylactic subtotal colectomy among hereditary nonpolyposis colorectal cancer germline mutation carriers? Dis Colon Rectum 1996;39:109–110.
73 Watson P, Vasen HF, Mecklin JP, Jarvinen H, Lynch HT: The risk of endometrial cancer in hereditary nonpolyposis colorectal cancer. Am J Med 1994;96:516–520.
74 Groden J, Thliveris A, Samowitz W, Carlson M, Gelbert L, Albertsen H, Joslyn G, Stevens J, Spirio L, Robertson M: Identification and characterization of the familial adenomatous polyposis coli gene. Cell 1991;66:589–600.
75 Ambroze WL Jr, Dozois RR, Pemberton JH, Beart RW Jr, Ilstrup DM: Familial adenomatous polyposis: Results following ileal pouch-anal anastomosis and ileorectostomy. Dis Colon Rectum 1992;35:12–15.
76 Madden MV, Neale KF, Nicholls RJ, Landgrebe JC, Chapman PD, Bussey HJ, Thomson JP: Comparison of morbidity and function after colectomy with ileorectal anastomosis or restorative proctocolectomy for familial adenomatous polyposis. Br J Surg 1991;78:789–792.
77 Nyam DC, Brillant PT, Dozois RR, Kelly KA, Pemberton JH, Wolff BG: Ileal pouch-anal canal anastomosis for familial adenomatous polyposis: Early and late results. Ann Surg 1997;226:514–519; discussion 519–521.
78 Heiskanen I, Matikainen M, Hiltunen K, Laitinen S, Rintala R, Jarvinen HJ: Colectomy and ileorectal anastomosis or restorative proctocolectomy for familial adenomatous polyposis. Colorectal Dis 1999;1:9–14.
79 Kartheuser AH, Parc R, Penna CP, Tiret E, Frileux P, Hannoun L, Nordlinger B, Loygue J: Ileal pouch-anal anastomosis as the first choice operation in patients with familial adenomatous polyposis: A ten-year experience. Surgery 1996;119:615–623.
80 Penna C, Tiret E, Kartheuser A, Hannoun L, Nordlinger B, Parc R: Function of ileal J pouch-anal anastomosis in patients with familial adenomatous polyposis. Br J Surg 1993;80:765–767.
81 Bulow C, Vasen H, Jarvinen H, Bjork J, Bisgaard ML, Bulow S: Ileorectal anastomosis is appropriate for a subset of patients with familial adenomatous polyposis. Gastroenterology 2000;119:1454–1460.
82 Vasen HF, van Duijvendijk P, Buskens E, Bulow C, Bjork J, Jarvinen JH, Bulow S: Decision analysis in the surgical treatment of patients with familial adenomatous polyposis: A Dutch-Scandinavian collaborative study including 659 patients. Gut 2001;49:231–235.
83 van Duijvendijk P, Vasen HF, Bertario L, Bulow S, Kuijpers JH, Schouten WR, Guillem JG, Taat CW, Slors JF: Cumulative risk of developing polyps or malignancy at the ileal pouch-anal anastomosis in patients with familial adenomatous polyposis. J Gastrointest Surg 1999;3:325–330.
84 Church JM, Oakley JR, Wu JS: Pouch polyposis after ileal pouch-anal anastomosis for familial adenomatous polyposis: Report of a case. Dis Colon Rectum 1996;39:584–586.
85 Nugent KP, Spigelman AD, Nicholls RJ, Talbot IC, Neale K, Phillips RK: Pouch adenomas in patients with familial adenomatous polyposis. Br J Surg 1993;80:1620.
86 Wu JS, McGannon EA, Church JM: Incidence of neoplastic polyps in the ileal pouch of patients with familial adenomatous polyposis after restorative proctocolectomy. Dis Colon Rectum 1998;41:552–556; discussion 556–557.
87 Heuschen UA, Heuschen G, Autschbach F, Allemeyer EH, Herfarth C: Adenocarcinoma in the ileal pouch: Late risk of cancer after restorative proctocolectomy. Int J Colorectal Dis 2001;16:126–130.

88 Parc YR, Olschwang S, Desaint B, Schmitt G, Parc RG, Tiret E: Familial adenomatous polyposis: Prevalence of adenomas in the ileal pouch after restorative proctocolectomy. Ann Surg 2001;233:360–364.
89 Milsom JW, Ludwig KA, Church JM, Garcia-Ruiz A: Laparoscopic total abdominal colectomy with ileorectal anastomosis for familial adenomatous polyposis. Dis Colon Rectum 1997;40:675–678.
90 Vasen HF, van der Luijt RB, Slors JF, Buskens E, de Ruiter P, Baeten CG, Schouten WR, Oostvogel HJ, Kuijpers JH, Tops CM, Meera Khan P: Molecular genetic tests as a guide to surgical management of familial adenomatous polyposis. Lancet 1996;348:433–435.
91 Marcello PW, Asbun HJ, Veidenheimer MC, Rossi RL, Roberts PL, Fine SN, Coller JA, Murray JJ, Schoetz DJ Jr: Gastroduodenal polyps in familial adenomatous polyposis. Surg Endosc 1996;10:418–421.
92 Burt RW, Berenson MM, Lee RG, Tolman KG, Freston JW, Gardner EJ: Upper gastrointestinal polyps in Gardner's syndrome. Gastroenterology 1984;86:295–301.
93 Bulow S, Lauritsen KB, Johansen A, Svendsen LB, Sondergaard JO: Gastroduodenal polyps in familial polyposis coli. Dis Colon Rectum 1985;28:90–93.
94 Jarvinen HJ, Sipponen P: Gastroduodenal polyps in familial adenomatous and juvenile polyposis. Endoscopy 1986;18:230–234.
95 Kurtz RC, Sternberg SS, Miller HH, Decosse JJ: Upper gastroinestinal neoplasia in familial polyposis. Dig Dis Sci 1987;32:459–465.
96 Sarre RG, Frost AG, Jagelman DG, Petras RE, Sivak MV, McGannon E: Gastric and duodenal polyps in familial adenomatous polyposis: A prospective study of the nature and prevalence of upper gastrointestinal polyps. Gut 1987;28:306–314.
97 Church JM, McGannon E, Hull-Boiner S, Sivak MV, Van Stolk R, Jagelman DG, Fazio VW, Oakley JR, Lavery IC, Milsom JW: Gastroduodenal polyps in patients with familial adenomatous polyposis. Dis Colon Rectum 1992;35:1170–1173.
98 Spigelman AD, Williams CB, Talbot IC, Domizio P, Phillips RK: Upper gastrointestinal cancer in patients with familial adenomatous polyposis. Lancet 1989;2:783–785.
99 Bulow S, Alm T, Fausa O, Hultcrantz R, Jarvinen H, Vasen H: Duodenal adenomatosis in familial adenomatous polyposis. DAF Project Group. Int J Colorectal Dis 1995;10:43–46.
100 Jagelman DG, DeCosse JJ, Bussey HJ: Upper gastrointestinal cancer in familial adenomatous polyposis. Lancet 1988;i:1149–1151.
101 Offerhaus GJ, Giardiello FM, Krush AJ, Booker SV, Tersmette AC, Kelley NC, Hamilton SR: The risk of upper gastrointestinal cancer in familial adenomatous polyposis. Gastronenterology 1992;102:1980–1982.
102 Vasen HF, Bulow S, Myrhoj T, Mathus-Vliegen L, Griffioen G, Buskens E, Taal BG, Nagengast F, Slors JF, de Ruiter P: Decision analysis in the management of duodenal adenomatosis in familial adenomatous polyposis. Gut 1997;40:716–719.
103 Penna C, Phillips RK, Tiret E, Spigelman AD: Surgical polypectomy of duodenal adenomas in familial adenomatous polyposis: Experience of two European centres. Br J Surg 1993;80:1027–1029.
104 Almy TP, Sherlock P: Genetic aspects of ulcerative colitis and regional enteritis. Gastroenterology 1966;51:757–763.
105 Kirsner JB: Genetic aspects of inflammatory bowel disease. Clin Gastroenterol 1973;21:557.
106 Ekbom A, Helmick C, Zack M, Adami HO: Ulcerative colitis and colorectal cancer. A population-based study. N Engl J Med 1990;323:1228–1233.
107 Gyde SN, Prior P, Allan RN, Stevens A, Jewell DP, Truelove SC, Lofberg R, Brostrom O, Hellers G: Colorectal cancer in ulcerative colitis: A cohort study of primary referrals from three centres. Gut 1988;29:206–217.
108 McDougall IPM: The cancer risk in ulcerative colitis. Lancet 1964;2:655–658.
109 Pinczowski D, Ekbom A, Baron J, Yuen J, Adami HO: Risk factors for colorectal cancer in patients with ulcerative colitis: A case-control study. Gastroenterology 1994;107:117–120.
110 Ohman U: Colorectal carcinoma in patients with ulcerative colitis. Am J Surg 1982;144:344–349.
111 Prior P, Gyde SN, Macartney JC, Thompson H, Waterhouse JA, Allan RN: Cancer morbidity in ulcerative colitis. Gut 1982;23:490–497.
112 Jayaram H, Satsangi J, Chapman RW: Increased colorectal neoplasia in chronic ulcerative colitis complicated by primary sclerosing cholangitis: Fact or fiction? Gut 2001;48:430–434.
113 Mir-Madjlessi SH, Farmer RG, Easley KA, Beck GJ: Colorectal and extracolonic malignancy in ulcerative colitis. Cancer 1986;58:1569–1574.
114 Devroede GJ, Taylor WF, Sauer WG, Jackman RJ, Stickler GB: Cancer risk and life expectancy of children with ulcerative colitis. N Engl J Med 1971;285:17–21.
115 Gorfine SR, Bauer JJ, Harris MT, Kreel I: Dysplasia complicating chronic ulcerative colitis: Is immediate colectomy warranted? Dis Colon Rectum 2000;43:1575–1581.
116 Johnson WR, McDermott FT, Pihl E, Hughes ES: Mucosal dysplasia. A major predictor of cancer following ileorectal anastomosis. Dis Colon Rectum 1983;26:697–700.
117 Gullberg K, Stahlberg D, Liljeqvist L, Tribukait B, Reinholt FP, Veress B, Lofberg R: Neoplastic transformation of the pelvic pouch mucosa in patients with ulcerative colitis. Gastroenterology 1997;112:1487–1492.
118 Nuako KW, Ahlquist DA, Mahoney DW, Schaid DJ, Siems DM, Lindor NM: Familial predisposition for colorectal cancer in chronic ulcerative colitis: A case-control study. Gastroenterology 1998;115:1079–1083.
119 Askling J, Dickman PW, Karlen P, Brostrom O, Lapidus A, Lofberg R, Ekbom A: Family history as a risk factor for colorectal cancer in inflammatory bowel disease. Gastroenterology 2001;120:1356–1362.
120 Brand RE, Lynch HT: Hereditary pancreatic adenocarcinoma. A clinical perspective. Med Clin North Am 2000;84:665–675.
121 Lal G, Liu G, Schmocker B, Kaurah P, Ozcelik H, Narod SA, Redston M, Gallinger S: Inherited predisposition to pancreatic adenocarcinoma: Role of family history and germline p16, BRCA1, and BRCA2 mutations. Cancer Res 2000;60:409–416.
122 Su GH, Hruban RH, Bansal RK, Bova GS, Tang DJ, Shekher MC, Westerman AM, Entius MM, Goggins M, Yeo CJ, Kern SE: Germline and somatic mutations of the STK11/LKB1 Peutz-Jeghers gene in pancreatic and biliary cancers. Am J Pathol 1999;154:1835–1840.
123 Whitcomb DC, Ulrich CD: Hereditary pancreatitis: New insights, new directions. Baillieres Best Pract Res Clin Gastroenterol 1999;13:253–263.
124 Brentnall TA: Cancer surveillance of patients from familial pancreatic cancer kindreds. Med Clin North Am 2000;84:707–718.
125 Bentjerodt R, Smok G: Ductal epithelial lesions and pancreatic adenocarcinoma. Rev Med Chil 1990;118:1099–1104.
126 Schulz HJ: Dysplasia and carcinoma in situ of the pancreatic duct epithelium. Zentralbl Allg Pathol 1988;134:3–14.
127 Cubilla AL, Fitzgerald PJ: Morphological lesions associated with human primary invasive nonendocrine pancreas cancer. Cancer Res 1976;36:2690–2698.
128 Kozuka S, Sassa R, Taki T, Masamoto K, Nagasawa S, Saga S, Hasegawa K, Takeuchi M: Relation of pancreatic duct hyperplasia to carcinoma. Cancer 1979;43:1418–1428.
129 Berberat P, Friess H, Kashiwagi M, Beger HG, Büchler MW: Diagnosis and staging of pancreatic cancer by positron emission tomography. World J Surg 1999;23:882–887.
130 Rosch T, Lorenz R, Braig C, Feuerbach S, Siewert JR, Schusdziarra V, Classen M: Endoscopic ultrasound in pancreatic tumor diagnosis. Gastrointest Endosc 1991;37:347–352.
131 Inokuma T, Tamaki N, Torizuka T, Magata Y, Fujii M, Yonekura Y, Kajiyama T, Ohshio G, Imamura M, Konishi J: Evaluation of pancreatic tumors with positron emission tomography and F-18 fluorodeoxyglucose: Comparison with CT and US. Radiology 1995;195:345–352.
132 Muller MF, Meyenberger C, Bertschinger P, Schaer R, Marincek B: Pancreatic tumors: Evaluation with endoscopic US, CT, and MR imaging. Radiology 1994;190:745–751.

133 Gress F, Gottlieb K, Cummings O, Sherman S, Lehman G: Endoscopic ultrasound characteristics of mucinous cystic neoplasms of the pancreas. Am J Gastroenterol 2000;95:961–965.

134 Gress F, Gottlieb K, Sherman S, Lehman G: Endoscopic ultrasonography-guided fine-needle aspiration biopsy of suspected pancreatic cancer. Ann Intern Med 2001;134:459–464.

135 Gress FG, Hawes RH, Savides TJ, Ikenberry SO, Cummings O, Kopecky K, Sherman S, Wiersema M, Lehman GA: Role of EUS in the preoperative staging of pancreatic cancer: A large single-center experience. Gastrointest Endosc 1999;50:786–791.

136 Taouli B, Vilgrain V, Vullierme MP, Terris B, Denys A, Sauvanet A, Hammel P, Menu Y: Intraductal papillary mucinous tumors of the pancreas: Helical CT with histopathologic correlation. Radiology 2000;217:757–764.

137 Ariyama J, Suyama M, Satoh K, Wakabayashi K: Endoscopic ultrasound and intraductal ultrasound in the diagnosis of small pancreatic tumors. Abdom Imaging 1998;23:380–386.

138 Friess H, Langhans J, Ebert M, Beger HG, Stollfuss J, Reske SN, Büchler MW: Diagnosis of pancreatic cancer by 2[^{18}F]-fluoro-2-deoxy-D-glucose positron emission tomography. Gut 1995;36:771–777.

139 Stollfuss JC, Glatting G, Friess H, Kocher F, Beger HG, Reske SN: 2-(fluorine-18)-fluoro-2-deoxy-D-glucose PET in detection of pancreatic cancer: Value of quantitative image interpretation. Radiology 1995;195:339–344.

140 Caldas C: Biliopancreatic malignancy: Screening the at risk patient with molecular markers. Ann Oncol 1999;10:153–156.

141 Terhune PG, Phifer DM, Tosteson TD, Longnecker DS: K-ras mutation in focal proliferative lesions of human pancreas. Cancer Epidemiol Biomarkers Prev 1998;7:515–521.

142 Lohr M, Maisonneuve P, Lowenfels AB: K-Ras mutations and benign pancreatic disease. Int J Pancreatol 2000;27:93–103.

143 Ritts RE, Pitt HA: CA 19-9 in pancreatic cancer. Surg Oncol Clin N Am 1998;7:93–101.

144 Brat DJ, Lillemoe KD, Yeo CJ, Warfield PB, Hruban RH: Progression of pancreatic intraductal neoplasias to infiltrating adenocarcinoma of the pancreas. Am J Surg Pathol 1998;22:163–169.

145 Hruban RH, Petersen GM, Goggins M, Tersmette AC, Offerhaus GJ, Falatko F, Yeo CJ, Kern SE: Familial pancreatic cancer. Ann Oncol 1999;10:69–73.

146 Goggins M, Canto M, Hruban R: Can we screen high-risk individuals to detect early pancreatic carcinoma? J Surg Oncol 2000;74:243–248.

147 Chen CH, Yang CC, Yeh YH, Chou DA, Kuo CL: Ectopic pancreas located in the major duodenal papilla: Case report and review. Gastrointest Endosc 2001;53:121–123.

148 Nagai H, Kuroda A, Morioka Y: Lymphatic and local spread of T1 and T2 pancreatic cancer. A study of autopsy material. Ann Surg 1986;204:65–71.

149 Seiler CA, Wagner M, Sadowski C, Kulli C, Büchler MW: Randomized prospective trial of pylorus-preserving vs. classic duodenopancreatectomy (Whipple procedure): Initial clinical results. J Gastrointest Surg 2000;4:443–452.

150 Wagner M, Dikopoulos N, Kulli C, Friess H, Büchler MW: Standard surgical treatment in pancreatic cancer. Ann Oncol 1999;10:247–251.

Original Paper

Digestive Diseases

Dig Dis 2002;20:102–105

Loss of Expression of Tumor Suppressor p16^{INK4} Protein in Human Primary Gastric Cancer Is Related to the Grade of Differentiation

Alba Rocco[a,b] Laslo Schandl[a,d] Gerardo Nardone[b] Zolt Tulassay[d]
Stefania Staibano[c] Peter Malfertheiner[a] Matthias P.A. Ebert[a]

[a]Department of Gastroenterology, Hepatology and Infectious Diseases, Otto-von-Guericke University, Magdeburg, Germany, [b]Department of Clinical and Experimental Medicine, Gastroenterology Unit, 'Federico II' University, and [c]Department of Pathology, 'Federico II' University, Naples, Italy, and [d]II Department of Internal Medicine, Semmelweis University, Budapest, Hungary

Key Words

p16 · Cell cycle inhibitors · Gastric cancer

Abstract

Background: Recent research has revealed a rapid increase in the number of alterations underlying oncogenesis and the proteins which regulate the cell cycle. p16 is a cell cycle regulatory protein acting as a cyclin-dependent kinase inhibitor (CDKI). Because of its antiproliferative effect, p16 has been suggested to be a tumor suppressor gene. Deletions, mutations and functional inactivation of p16 occur with a frequency second only to p53 in most human malignancies. ***Aim:*** to evaluate the p16 protein expression in primary gastric cancer in order to understand the possible differences in relation to histotype and grade of tumors. ***Material and Methods:*** Immunohistochemical expression of p16 was investigated in matched normal and cancerous tissues from 70 patients with gastric cancer (52 intestinal and 18 diffuse type). ***Results:*** In non-cancerous gastric tissues the immunostaining of p16 was weak and limited to antral glands. In gastric cancer tissues, the enhanced immunoreactivity of p16 was not significantly different in intestinal and diffuse type of gastric cancer. However, the intensity of immunostaining was inversely related to the grade of differentiation of these tumours. ***Conclusions:*** The overexpression of p16 seems to be a common event in the development of both intestinal and diffuse type of gastric cancer and it is likely that it may be driven by features of the neoplastic state. Likewise, the absence of p16 in the lowest grade of differentiation may reflect increased selection pressure and clonal expansion of the cells with a more aggressive phenotype.

Supported by the DAAD, DFG and Land Sachsen-Anhalt.

Introduction

The p16^{INK4} gene codes for a cyclin-dependent kinase inhibitory protein which acts as a major tumor suppressor. The p16 gene has been found to be altered in several human malignancies at a frequency rivaling the p53 gene [1]. The alterations frequently involving the p16 gene have been grouped in three distinct classes: sequence changes in genomic DNA such as point mutations or small deletions [2]; homozygous deletions of long segments of DNA that include p16 [3]; and transcriptional suppression of p16 by methylation of the promoter region and exon 1 [4, 5]. The last mechanism seems to be of

KARGER

Fax + 41 61 306 12 34
E-Mail karger@karger.ch
www.karger.com

0257–2753/02/0201–0102$18.50/0

Accessible online at:
www.karger.com/journals/ddi

M.P.A. Ebert, MD
Department of Gastroenterology, Hepatology and Infectious Diseases
Otto-von-Guericke University, Leipzigerstrasse 44, D–39120 Magdeburg (Germany)
Tel. +49 391 6713156, Fax +49 391 67190054
E-Mail Matthias.Ebert@medizin.uni-magdeburg.de

major importance for p16 inactivation in human gastric carcinoma [6]. In any case the inactivation of the p16 gene shows strong correlation with the loss of immunoreactivity for the p16 protein [7].

In this light we examined the p16 protein expression in matched normal and cancerous tissues from patients with gastric cancer in order to understand the possible differences or relations of the p16 immuno-pattern with type and grade of differentiation of primary human gastric cancers.

Materials and Methods

Tissue Samples

Tissue samples for immunohistochemical analysis were collected from patients who underwent gastric cancer surgery. The study population consisted of 70 patients, 50 men, 20 women. The mean age was 59.9 years (SD: 10.6 years, range: 26–86 years). This study was approved by the Ethics Committee of the University of Magdeburg.

Histology

According to the histological growth pattern [8], we classified the carcinoma tissues into intestinal and diffuse type of tumor. There were 52 carcinomas of the intestinal type and 18 carcinomas of the diffuse type. The grade of differentiation was poor in 41 gastric cancer, moderate in 23 and well differentiated in 6 tumors. The tumors were confined to the mucosa or submucosa in 2 cases (all of the intestinal type) and advanced in 68 cases.

Immunohistochemistry

Sections (4 μm) were dewaxed and rehydrated, then the endogenous peroxidase activity was inhibited by incubation with 0.3% H_2O_2-methanol solution (30 min at room temperature). To enhance immunostaining sections were heated two times in a microwave oven at high power. Antigen retrieval was performed with 0.1 *M* trinatriumcitrate dihydrate, pH 6.0, 0.1 *M* citric acid solution.

To reduce non-specific background staining slides were incubated with normal goat serum for 20 min at room temperature. Finally, the slides were incubated with the appropriate primary antisera in humidity chambers over night at 4 °C. The primary polyclonal antibody used was anti-p16 (15126 PharMingen, San Diego; Calif.) at a dilution of 1:100. Detection of the bound primary antibody was performed using the standard HRP-Streptavidin System (Kirkegaard & Perry Laboratories USA). Peroxidase activity was detected with diaminobenzidine as substrate. Finally, the slides were weakly counterstained with haematoxylin and mounted with a mounting medium.

Furthermore, to ensure the specificity of immunostaining we performed immunohistochemistry using consecutive sections in the absence of the primary antibody and with preimmune serum. In all of these cases no immunostaining was detected.

The degree of immunopositivity was evaluated semiquantitatively. The number of positive cells was counted and expressed as percentages. The immunoreactivity was graded as negative (0–5%), low positivity (5–25%), moderate positivity (25–50%), and high positivity (>50%).

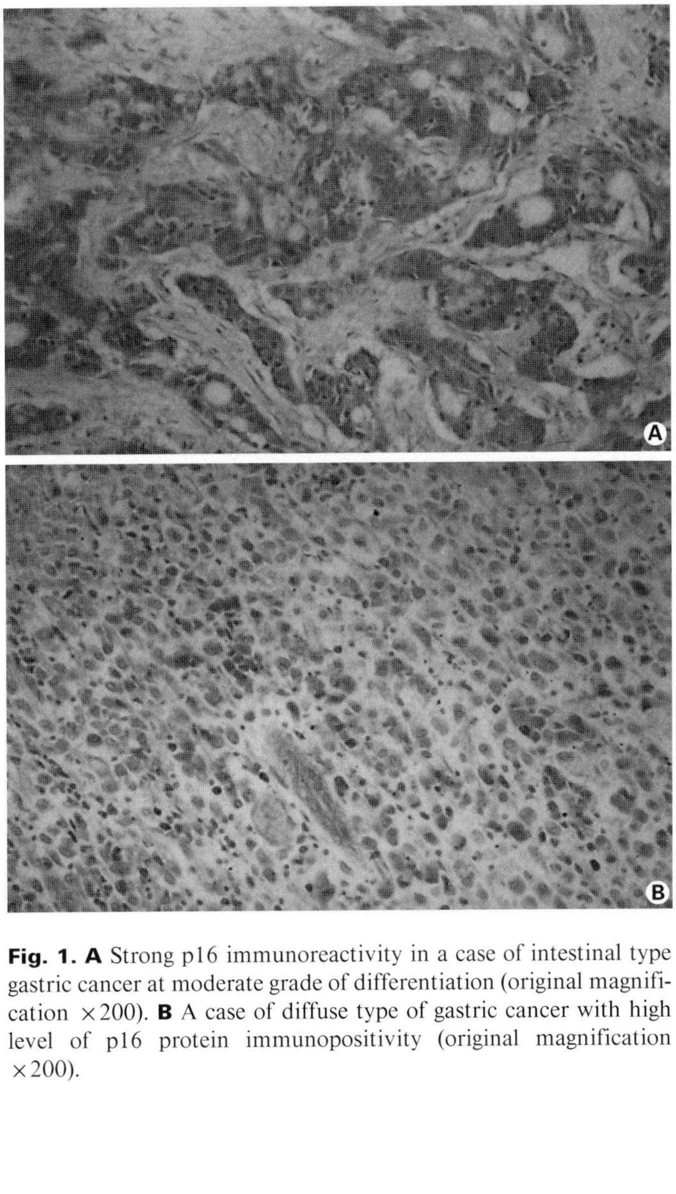

Fig. 1. A Strong p16 immunoreactivity in a case of intestinal type gastric cancer at moderate grade of differentiation (original magnification ×200). **B** A case of diffuse type of gastric cancer with high level of p16 protein immunopositivity (original magnification ×200).

Statistical Analysis

The different expression of p16 protein in relation to histotype and grade of differentiation was determined by Fisher's exact test. Spearman test was used to evaluate the correlation of p16 expression with the grade of differentiation of the cancers. A p value <0.05 was taken as the level of significance.

Results

In non-neoplastic gastric mucosa the immunostaining of p16 was weak and selectively distributed in the antral glands.

In the gastric cancer p16 was overexpressed in 71% of the cases with strong immunoreactivity in 42% of the cancers (fig. 1A, B) but the overexpression of this protein was

Table 1. Immunohistochemical expression of p16 protein in relation to histotype of gastric cancer

	Intestinal type*	Diffuse type*	Total
p16 negative	13 (19%)	7 (10%)	20 (29%)
p16 positive	39 (56%)	11 (16%)	50 (71%)
Total	52 (74%)	18 (26%)	70 (100%)

* p = 0.3641 (Fisher's exact test).

Table 2. Correlation of p16 and grade of differentiation of tumors

	p16 expression*			
	–	+	++	+++
Well	0	0	0	8 (100%)
Moderate	0	4 (19%)	9 (43%)	8 (38%)
Poor	9 (22%)	25 (61%)	6 (15%)	1 (2%)

* Spearman r = –0.6641; p < 0.0001; –/+++ intensity of immunostaining.

not significantly different in relation to the histotype of gastric cancer (table 1).

Furthermore, the intensity of immunostaining of p16 was directly related to the grade of differentiation of the tumours (table 2): p16 immunoreactivity was significantly lower in poorly differentiated than in well or moderately differentiated adenocarcinomas ($p < 0.001$).

Discussion

Gastric cancer may be considered the final step of a progressive imbalance between mucosal cell proliferation and apoptosis due to the activation of oncogenes and the inactivation of tumor suppressor genes [9, 10].

p16 is a cell-cycle regulatory protein acting as a cyclin-dependent kinase inhibitor. Because of its antiproliferative effect, p16 has been suggested to be a tumor suppressor gene. Deletions, mutations and functional inactivation involve the p16 gene with a frequency second only to p53 in most human malignancies [1]. However, the transcriptional suppression of p16 by methylation of the promoter region and exon 1 seems to be the major mechanism of p16 inactivation in human gastric carcinoma [4–6]. In any case, the inactivation of p16 gene shows strong correlation with the tissue immunoreactivity for the p16 protein [7].

In this light we examined the immunohistochemical expression of the p16 protein in tumoral and non tumoral mucosa of seventy patients with primary gastric cancers.

In the normal mucosa we found weak immunopositivity restricted to antral glands. In contrast, tumoral areas exhibited p16 overexpression in the majority of the cases (fig. 1A, B). These results confirm the notion derived from in vitro experiments that p16 may be induced by oncogenic events [12].

The frequency of the overexpression of this protein was not significantly different between the two histological types, intestinal and diffuse, of gastric cancer (table 1). However, there was a strong association between p16 overexpression and a higher histological grade of differentiation (table 2).

Taken together, these data suggest that the overexpression of p16 is not typical for a specific pathway for the development of the two main histological types of gastric cancer. However, it seems to be a common event in the development of both intestinal and diffuse types of gastric cancer.

Likewise, the significant relation between loss or weak expression of p16 and poorly differentiated cancers may reflect an increased selection pressure and clonal expansion of the cells in which p16 expression has been suppressed and, thus, which may exhibit a more aggressive phenotype.

Acknowledgements

We thank Frau Ingrid Bierwirth for providing excellent technical assistance.

References

1 Kamb A, Gruis NA, Weaver-Feldhaus J, Liu Q, Harshman K, Tavtigian SV, et al: A cell cycle regulator potentially involved in genesis of many tumor types. Science 1994;264:436–440.

2 Pollock PM, Pearson JV, Hayward NK: Compilation of somatic mutations of the CDKN2 gene in human cancers: non-random distribution of base substitutions. Genes Chromosomes Cancer 1996;15(2):77–88.

3 Stone S, Jiang P, Dayananth P, Tavtigian SV, Katcher H, Parry D, et al: Complex structure and regulation of the P16 (MTS1) locus. Cancer Res 1995;55(14):2988–2994.

4 Merlo A, Herman JG, Mao L, Lee DJ, Gabrielson E, Burger PC, et al: 5′ CpG island methylation is associated with transcriptional silencing of the tumour suppressor p16/CDKN2/MTS1 in human cancers. Nat Med 1995; 1(7):686–692.

5 Otterson GA, Khleif SN, Chen W, Coxon AB, Kaye FJ: CDKN2 gene silencing in lung cancer by DNA hypermethylation and kinetics of p16INK4 protein induction by 5-aza 2′deoxycytidine. Oncogene 1995;11(6):1211–1216.

6 Lee YY, Kang SH, Seo JY, Jung CW, Lee KU, Choe KJ, et al: Alterations of p16INK4A and p15INK4B genes in gastric carcinomas. Cancer 1997;80(10):1889–1896.

7 Shim YH, Kang GH, Ro JY. Correlation of p16 hypermethylation with p16 protein loss in sporadic gastric carcinomas. Lab Invest 2000; 80(5):689–695.

8 Lauren P: The two histological main types of gastric carcinoma: diffuse and so-called intestinal-type carcinoma. Acta Path Microbiol Scand 1995;64:31–49.

9 Correa P, Shiao YH: Phenotypic and genotypic events in gastric carcinogenesis. Cancer Res 1994;54(suppl 7):1941s–1943s.

10 Farber E: Cancer development and its natural history. A cancer prevention perspective. Cancer 1988;62(suppl 8):1676–1679.

11 Farber E: Reversible and irreversible lesions in processes of cancer development. IARC Sci Publ 1980;(27):143–151.

12 Serrano M, Lin AW, McCurrach ME, Beach D, Lowe SW: Oncogenic ras provokes premature cell senescence associated with accumulation of p53 and p16^{INK4a}. Cell 1997;88:593–602.

Digestive Diseases

Author Index Vol. 20, No. 1, 2002

Subject Index Vol. 20, No. 1, 2002

KARGER
Fax +41 61 306 12 34
E-Mail karger@karger.ch
www.karger.com

Accessible online at:
www.karger.com/journals/ddi